Promoting the Health of School Age Children

Promoting the Health of School Age Children

Edited by
Jane Wright
and
Val Thurtle

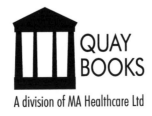

QUAY
BOOKS

A division of MA Healthcare Ltd

Quay Books Division, MA Healthcare Ltd, St Jude's Church, Dulwich Road, London
SE24 0PB

British Library Cataloguing-in-Publication Data
A catalogue record is available for this book

© MA Healthcare Limited 2008. Reprint 2010

ISBN-10: 1 85642 356 5
ISBN-13: 978 1 85642 356 4

Printed by CLE Group Ltd, Media House, Burrel Road, St Ives, Cambridgeshire PE27 3LE.

Contents

Contents

Foreword

In the increasingly complex world of changing family structures, advancing technologies and changes to the ethnic structures of the population in many of our cities, it comes as no surprise that the role of children's nurses in the future will need to adapt and respond innovatively to the challenges this presents.

School nurses will clearly take a lead in health needs assessment, working strategically at population level to ensure that service provision across health, education and local authorities meets the needs of our children. Some will lead teams of integrated children's workers, whereas others will be working at the front line with children from some of the most vulnerable families, requiring skills to negotiate and develop trusting relationships that in turn will improve the long-term outcomes for the most socially excluded families.

The Chief Nursing Officer's review of school nursing in 2006 identified the modernised role for school nurses and this set the precedent to raise the profile of school nursing and the unique added value they bring to the public's health. What it also introduced, which has been supported by further policy drivers, is the idea of an integrated children's workforce across health education and local authorities. Alongside this is the introduction of skill mix and the view of the school nurse as a team leader. This for some is quite a significant shift from current practice, where they have been working single-handed as the health practitioner in a school setting, often marginalised but nonetheless making a significant difference to the children and the families they work with.

Community children's nurses will be working with children with increasingly complex health needs in the community, from acute illness to managing children with long-term illnesses and in the terminal phase of their life. This will present challenges, but it will also offer rewarding experiences for all concerned. In doing so the needs of the workforce must not be lost in service provision, in providing support and supervision relevant to need.

The recent review of the role of the health visitor, *Facing the Future: a Review of the Role of Health Visitors* (2007) has identified two key roles, one of leading the child health promotion programme and secondly working with the most challenging families and utilising their specialist skills to improve health outcome. Although not explicit, this model applies as much to the roles of the school nurse as to that of the health visitor, and indeed children's needs persist into school years and are often the most pertinent at times of transition. This message is clearly being relayed by many commissioners of children's services as they look at commissioning a 0–19 pathway and see children along a continuum.

In response to the shift in philosophy, it is anticipated that proposed changes in education and training will reflect the competencies required in delivering shifting political agendas that improve the health and well-being of the school aged population. These will be considered along the continuum of 0–19 years, focusing on parenting, behavioural therapies, emotional health and well-being, and public health priorities.

As increasingly more children are diagnosed with autistic spectrum disorders and behavioural conditions, more nurses with the skills to work long term with these children and their families will be needed, as will those working in the field of learning disability.

Any text on promoting the health of school age children and young people is faced with the challenges that the devolved government administrations across the United Kingdom pose. They all have similar challenges in addressing the health needs of the school age population in an increasingly complex society; however, how they choose to address these will be down to local determination. This book will provide school nurses and others with an excellent resource to make sense of the changing political agenda and the context for contemporary practice in addressing public health priorities. The content will prepare those who work with children and their families to make a real difference to the health outcomes of the school age child, enabling them to meet their real potential wherever they live across the UK.

Liz Plastow
Professional Advisor Specialist Community Public Health Nursing

Biographies

Joanne Bartley
Route Leader for School Nursing, Liverpool John Moores University
Joanne began her school nursing career sixteen years ago, as a caseload holder in a semi-rural area. She then moved to the Health Authority to work as a Health Promotion Specialist for Schools, specialising in sex and drugs education. Whilst undertaking a Masters degree in health promotion she seized the chance to become the Course Leader for School Nursing at Leeds Metropolitan University. She has worked at the University of Central Lancashire, the University of Leeds and is currently route leader for school nursing at Liverpool John Moores University.

Gill Coverdale
Senior Lecturer, Community Public Health Nursing, Leeds Metropolitan University
Gill has been nursing since 1980 and became a school nurse in 1988. She was responsible for setting up 'Walk in services for children and young people' in her local town. She came into education in 1999, working first in the further education sector as a lecturer/practitioner before moving into higher education. Gill has a passion for promoting and maintaining the mental and emotional well-being of children and families and has also written on parenting the adolescent.

Pat Day
Senior Lecturer in Primary Care Nursing , Sheffield Hallam University
Pat is part of the community nursing team at Sheffield Hallam University. She worked in Sheffield as a school nurse team leader, practice teacher and family planning nurse. Her interests include young people's sexual health. As part of a multi-agency team, Pat set up one of the first sexual health clinics on the site of a school.

Penny Farrelly
Senior Lecturer in Public health, Bucks New University

After practising as a Health Visitor Penny moved into education as a senior lecturer in public health and primary care, teaching student health visitors, community nurses and school nurses at BSc and MSc levels. She is currently involved in a research project looking at the ways in which pre-registration nurses develop their knowledge of public health. She is also involved in developing and coordinating a range of Foundation Degrees aimed at people working in early years and child settings.

Ros Godson
Community Practitioners' and Health Visitors' Association/Unite

Ros comes from a School Nursing background and is currently professional officer for school health and public health with the Community Practitioners' and Health Visitors' Association/Unite.

Maxine Jameson
Course Director School Nursing, London South Bank University

Maxine is passionate about the health and well-being of children and young people and has been a community nurse for the past 12 years. Maxine has worked in health, education, social services and for the Department of Health; she currently runs the specialist community public health nursing (school nursing) programme at London South Bank University.

Liz Numadi
Senior Lecturer in Child Health, Bucks New University

Liz is a children's nurse who has worked within the specialism of paediatric gastroenterology, supporting children and families with complex needs. She currently works as a nurse lecturer providing education for pre- and post-registration children's nurses, often with a focus on children with lifelong or chronic disease.

Kate Potter
Senior Lecturer and Course Leader Specialist Community Public Health Nursing, Bucks New University

Coming from children's nursing, Kate qualified as a health visitor 16 years ago. Having worked in practice she is now in higher education. Her main role is with Specialist Community Public Health Nursing and she has a special interest in the role of the community practitioner in Child Protection.

Elizabeth Joy Power
Course Director, Specialist Community Public Health Nursing, London South Bank University
Joy comes from a health visiting and community practice teaching background and now teaches at foundation, BSc and MSc level. She has previously facilitated Positive-Parenting Programmes and a Dyspraxia Support Group for parents. She has been a Sunday school teacher for 15 years and has assisted with Church Youth Group Activities.

Sarah Sherwin
Senior Lecturer University of Wolverhampton
Sarah Sherwin is a senior lecturer and course leader for school nursing at the University of Wolverhampton. In 1996 she was awarded a first class honours degree in school nursing and has subsequently gained a MA in Education. Sarah has been involved in school nursing since 1986 and has represented school nurses at a national level. She is currently Chair of the National Forum of School Health Educators.

Elaine Tabony
School Health Team Leader, Hillingdon Primary Care Trust
Elaine trained as a paediatric nurse at Great Ormond Street Hospital and practised in acute paediatrics before working as a school nurse and then as a team leader. Elaine received a Queen's Nursing Institute Award as project lead to establish the Seasons for Growth Grief Education Programme in Hillingdon. She leads the Community Nurse Continuing Professional Development programme for Personal Social Health Education in Hillingdon. Elaine led a pilot project for the M.E.N.D. programme tackling childhood obesity.

Val Thurtle
Senior Lecturer, University of Greewich
Coming from a health visiting background Val now works in education. She was previously a Programme Director Public Health Nursing at the University of Reading. She has taught nursery nurses, early childhood studies undergraduates, school nurses health visitors and community nurses. Over the years she has been involved in scouts, has taught at Sunday school and has been a school governor. Research interests have focused on career trajectories and identity in relation to community and public health nurses.

Alison Williams

School Nurse Team Leader Worcestershire/Part-time Senior Lecturer in Primary Care, University of Wolverhampton

Alison has been a school nurse professional advisor and has a degree in school nursing. Alison is currently studying for a Masters degree in clinical practice.

Jane Wright

Senior Lecturer in Public Health and Child Studies, Bucks New University

Jane teaches on a range of programmes related to children and young people, including Foundation, BSc and MSc levels. She worked as a community school nurse for six years and was influential in setting up multi-agency school-based health services in South Buckinghamshire. She has a keen interest in the health behaviours of adolescents and she has been involved in research exploring young people's attitudes to alcohol in Buckinghamshire.

Abbreviations

AIDS	Acquired Immunodeficiency Syndrome
CAMHS	Child and Adolescent Mental Health Service
CBT	Cognitive Behavioural Therapy
CHPP	Child Health Promotion Programme
CIPW	Creating an Interprofessional Workforce
CWDC	Children's Workforce Development Council
DCSF	Department for Children, Schools and Families
DCMS	Department for Culture Media and Sport
DH	Department of Health
DfES	Department for Education and Skills
DfEE	Department for Education and Employment
DRC	Disability Rights Commission
DWP	Department for Work and Pensions
ECM	Every Child Matters
FNN	Family Nurturing Network
HDA	Health Development Agency
HIV	Human Immunodeficiency Virus
LLI	Life Limiting Illnesses
M.E.N.D.	Mind, Exercise, Nutrition, Do it!
NCB	National Children's Bureau
NFPI	National Families and Parenting Institute
NHSP	National Healthy School Programme
NICE	National Institute of Clinical Health Excellence
NSF	National Service Framework
NSM	National Social Marketing
NSPCC	Nation Society for the Prevention of Cruelty to Children
NMC	Nursing and Midwifery Council
OCD	Obsessive Compulsive Disorder
OFSTED	Office for Standards in Education,Children's Services and Skills
PSHE	Personal Social and Health Education
QCA	Qualifications and Curriculum Authority
SCPHN	Specialist Community Public Health Nurse
SEF	Self Evaluation Forms
SEU	Social Exclusion Unit
SRE	Sex and Relationship Education

STI	Sexually Transmitted Infections
TUC	Trade Union Congress
UNICEF	United Nations Children's Fund
WHO	World Health Organization
ZPD	Zone of Proximinal Development

Introduction

Val Thurtle and Jane Wright

This book, as the title says, is about the health of the school-aged child and explores health in its widest sense, which could cover anything and everything related to the child or young person.

A classic and much used definition of health is:

A state of complete physical, mental and social well-being and not merely the absence of disease (WHO, 1946).

While this definition can be criticised, it is a starting point for this book, which considers ways of achieving optimum health for children and young people in all circumstances. This text is concerned with examining the promotion of the physical, mental and social well-being of children and young people. It aims to discuss some, but not all, of the factors that influence this well-being and in particular how those working with children can promote their health.

Children have always been important to their own parents, who generally want to do the best for their own child. Parents in different times and places may have had differing views as to what the best is, and have brought their children up in very diverse ways. The State became interested in children through the 19th and early 20th centuries, developing universal education, health care and social care for those whose parents could not provide appropriately for them. While provision for children and young people dates back over a hundred years, some may feel that concern has often been focused on the very young child in terms of health and the adolescent in terms of potential difficulties. The school-aged child is often only discussed in terms of educational achievement and not the relationship between health and well-being and the potential to learn. Much has been written about multidisciplinary working, but the extent to which services for children and young people have been integrated and how well health, education and care work together can be questioned.

If State services for children have been provided for some years and inter-agency working has long been advocated, one might ask why children and young people are high on today's agenda and why the development of this text is needed now.

In the past, concerns for children's health might have focused on survival rates and the number of children living in poverty, but statistics demonstrate a clear improvement in both infant and child mortality rates and those living in poverty in the UK. While these remain concerns in terms of inequalities, there are other public anxieties around children and young people often fuelled by frenetic media coverage. Are children being properly prepared for their future? Is their education appropriate and of a sufficiently high standard? Are children out of control? Is modern parenting an issue? Is their health good enough for now and are they laying down difficulties for the future?

On a community level there has been discussion as to whether there are sufficient children to become a workforce able to sustain an older population. Questions have been articulated as to whether their upbringing and education provide them with the educational skills for the workforce of tomorrow. In terms of health and upbringing, the precursors of limited exercise and a poor diet in childhood may facilitate obesity and its health effects, reducing life expectancy and making heavy demands on the health services of the future. Styles of parenting and stressors impacting on mental health may, too, have large-scale consequences for the adults of the future.

On a more individual level it is not difficult to find examples of children and young people as 'problems', having behaviour difficulties, being involved in crime, becoming pregnant or developing dependence on alcohol or drugs. Such issues present difficulties here and now, worrying parents and calling on police, social care, educational and health resources.

For most children and young people, care and protection are the priority. For many children life is good: they have caring parents, a secure upbringing, and access to good schools, health care and leisure facilities. Others do not have good relationships with those who care for them, live in poverty and use health and educational services that could be better. These inequalities may go on quietly, but occasionally a child hits the news with a 'disaster' story. Those who have worked with children for some years could name several such stories. The most recent and shocking was the death of Victoria Climbié, an eight-year-old girl who, in 2000, was abused, tortured and eventually killed by her great aunt and the man with whom they lived. The United Nations adopted the Convention on the Rights of the Child in 1989 (United Nations, 1989), which stated that the child (any person under the age of 18), requires special protection in order to develop his or her full potential, free from hunger and want, neglect, exploitation or other abuses. By 2007, 140 signatories, including the United Kingdom, had ratified the Convention on the Rights of the Child (OUNHCHR, 2007). In the UK, the Laming Report (2003), investigating Victoria's death, among other enquiries, acted as a catalyst to concentrate people's attention more effectively on the safety of vulnerable children, placing children high on the public agenda. The concerns were strongly influential in the development of the government green paper *Every Child Matters* (DfES/DH, 2003) and prompted unprecedented debate about services for children, young people and their families.

The document, which was given legal status in the form of the Children Act 2004 (DH, 2004), made it clear that it is everyone's responsibility to help achieve the five key outcomes for all children. The outcomes were for children and young people to:

- Be healthy
- Stay safe
- Enjoy and achieve
- Make a positive contribution
- Achieve economic well-being

The five outcomes are central to government policy and have been transferred into other documents and initiatives such as the National Service Framework for Children, Young People and Maternity Service (DH/DfES, 2004), Youth Matters (DfES, 2005), Extended Schools and Children's Centres (DfES, 2006a) and the Common Assessment Framework (DfES, 2006b), and it forms the basis for the Children's Plan: Building brighter futures (DCSF, 2007).

The five outcomes from *Every Child Matters* are central to this book and are alluded to in most chapters. Readers will find out about the child and young person and examine some of the policies mentioned. Most important is the outworking of the policies: how practitioners of all types can facilitate the promotion of health for and with children and young people.

Most of the contributors, and many of the expected readers, are from traditional health backgrounds, but health is too important to be left to health workers alone. School nurses, children's nurses, teachers, mental health workers, social workers, youth workers, care managers and others all need to be involved in the outworking of policies that promote health in its widest sense. The health and development of children have always been important for those working with children and young people. To go beyond this and to work towards genuine inter-agency holistic partnerships with children and young people, with more 'joined up thinking' between agencies, both statutory and voluntary, needs cultural change. To achieve this, there is an expectation that all those working with children and young people will be trained to a national standard as part of an overall children's workforce strategy and that this training will be across sectors (HM Government, 2005; DfES, 2006c). This book aims to be a resource for that workforce which explores the knowledge and skills required to improve the outcomes for children and young people outlined in Every Child Matters.

References

Department for Children, Schools and Families (2007) The *Children's Plan*. DCSF, London.

Department for Education and Skills (2005) *Youth Matters: Next Steps – Something to Do, Somewhere to Go, Someone to Talk to*. DfES Publications, Nottingham.

Department for Education and Skills (2006a) *The Common Assessment Framework: Practitioners' Guide*. Stationery Office, London.

Department for Education and Skills (2006b) *The Governance and Management of Extended Schools and Sure Start Children's Centres*. DfES, Nottingham.

Department for Education and Skills (2006c) *Children's Workforce Strategy: Building an Integrated Qualifications Framework*. DfES, London.

Department of Health/Department for Education and Skills (DH/DfES) (2003) *Every Child Matters*. Stationery Office, London.

Department of Health (2004) *The Children Act*. DH, London.

Department of Health and Department for Education and Skills (2004) *National Service Framework for Children, Young People and Maternity Services*. Stationery Office, London.

HM Government (2005) *Common Core of Skills and Knowledge for the Children's Workforce*. DfES, London.

Laming, Lord (2003) *The Victoria Climbié Inquiry: Report of an Inquiry by Lord Laming*. Stationery Office, London.

Office of the United Nations High Commission for Human Rights (OUNHCHR) (2007) *Convention on the Rights of the Child*. http://www2.ohchr.org/english/law/crc.htm; accessed 4 February 2008.

United Nations (1989) *Convention on the Rights of the Child*. http://www2.ohchr.org/english/law/crc.htm; accessed 4 February 2008.

World Health Organisation (1946) *Constitution*. World Health Organization, Geneva.

CHAPTER 1

Children and young people: what are they like?

Val Thurtle

Key themes

- Examination of different views of children and young people
- Broad outline of their physical development
- Introduction to different psychological perspectives
- Reflection on diverse constructions of childhood

Introduction

Children and young people are high on the political agenda and much discussed in the media. We may feel that we have a clear and shared idea of what a child is, yet this chapter will explore different views of children. While there are patterns as to how they develop, there are differences between individual children and enormous diversity in how they are viewed in different times and in different cultures.

This text places the focus on children and young people between 5 and 16 years of age who, at least in the United Kingdom context, are expected to be receiving education. Yet with the growth in nursery education and the development of the Early Years Foundation Stage (Department for Education and Skills [DfES], 2007) of the National Curriculum, the child is influenced by the education system at an earlier age. Sixteen is currently the end of compulsory education, but by 1999, 76% were remaining in education in schools, further education or higher education to a later stage (Office for National Statistics [ONS], 2002). The age of the end of compulsory education may well change, as a consultation is under way (Department for Children, Schools and Families [DCSF], 2007), with a plan to raise the school leaving age in England by 2013.

With these changes taking place even the definition of the school-aged child is barely a fixed point.

While this is occurring in the 21st century, there has been change over time. The end of compulsory school was 11 years of age in 1893 and had risen to 16 by 1972, though whether all children attended all the time is another issue. Different individuals and parts of society have demonstrated their different desires for, and expectations of, the child, which is not only demonstrated in terms of education but also ideas on childhood, child rearing, learning, parenting and more. This can all be seen as cultural relativism, which Stainton-Rogers (2001, p. 26) suggests is constructed by the 'human meaning makers'. These meaning makers might come from the media, church, politics, education or elsewhere and influence the dominant concept of the child and how he or she should be treated.

Even if the view of the child has changed over time, surely one could argue that the child or young person is a physical entity that would be much the same, whether considered in the United Kingdom today, elsewhere in the world or at some other point in history. The answer to this is probably not. Human bodies may work in the same way, but a variety of physical, environmental and social factors act upon children, leading to great differences and diversity in the world of the child, in which we can, at best, trace patterns rather than identify fixed attributes.

Those working with children and young people should be aware of different perspectives taken on children and seek to take a holistic view. In considering different aspects of the child it is useful to see the child and young person under particular headings, namely physical, psychological and social.

Physical

The biological characteristics of a child or young person might be seen as the most precise. The human body is made up of the same anatomical parts and each child learns to run, jump, read, write and do arithmetic within his or her capability. Yet a quick reflection should lead to the observation that some are taller than others, jump higher and are more able at the academic activities.

Using educational terms of Key Stages 1–4 (first introduced in the Education Reform Act 1988, but now routinely used) it is worth considering what these children and young people are like and what they can do. A starting framework is provided in Tables 1.1–1.3. It is however only a starting point and anyone who has had any contact with a child or young person between 5 and 18 will find statements included that they want to refine or even rewrite.

Reflection on the figures leads to the observation that there is great variation in height, running and reading skills, language development and interaction with others, and empirical research bears this out. There is therefore a

Table 1.1 An approximate guide to development in children: Key Stage 1 – child 5–7 years old.

Physical attributes		Weight	Height	
	Girls	12–32 kg	100–134 cm	There are wide ranges and rapid growth spurts take place
	Boys	15–31 kg	101–135cm	
	Weights and heights alone mean little, but should be plotted on a centile chart (Child Growth Development Foundation, 1996)			
	85–90% 5–7-year-olds dry by night			
Gross motor	Hops on either foot			Tip toes
	Walks up and down stairs one foot per step			Increasing skills of climbing, kicking, throwing and catching ball
	Skips			Confident and competent in movements
	Walks along line			
	Rides two-wheeler bike			
Fine motor	Writes letters of name and goes on to write words with concentration			Can dress and undress
	Uses large needle			Uses knife and fork
	Threads beads well			Ties bow
	Hold pencil tripod style			Uses scissors
				Can draw □ or △ by 7; copies
Cognitive and language	Conversation developing, clear to those outside usual contacts			Begins to see the world in terms of rules
	Rate of vocabulary varies but may have 15,000 words, gaining 3,000 per year			Thinking generally related to specific experiences
	Some substitutions still in evidence e.g. 'f' for 'th'			Beginning to use simple logic
	By 7 understands and uses conjunctions, tag questions, passive tense and infinitives			By 7 able to categorise items, e.g. dinosaurs, football teams
				Using number and learning to tell time
				Has simple concepts of distance, time and speed
Social emotional and behavioural	Cooperative play, sharing toys			Play tends to be with children of same sex
	Rough and tumble play			Segregates into gender groups
	Socio-dramatic play			Discovering importance of friends, may have 'best friend'
	Plays games with increasingly complicated rules			
	Protective towards younger siblings			

Table 1.2 An approximate guide to development in children: Key Stage 2 – child 7–11 years old.

Physical attributes	Girls	Weight	16–55 kg	Height	111–157 cm	There are wide ranges and rapid growth spurts take place
	Boys		16–52 kg		112–157 cm	
	Weights and heights alone mean little, but should be plotted on a centile chart (Child Growth Development Foundation, 1996)					
	Head and brain fully grown, long bones and trunk lengthen					
	95% 10-year-olds have bladder control, but boys are over represented in those not dry by night					
Gross motor	Strength and agility and coordination developing					
	Increased speed in running and accuracy in throwing and kicking ball					
	Many play in team sport ,though there are concerns about the amount of exercise taken (DH, 2004)					
Fine motor	Increasing coordination, writing and drawing, musical instruments, model making, keyboard skills					
	Potential to develop embroidery and carving skills					
Cognitive	Beginning to see and understand others' points of view					
	Increasing complexity of language and number of words					
	Developing syntax (grammar)					
	Using and understanding conjunctions, tag questions, passive tenses and infinitives					
Social emotional and behavioural	Friendship based on reciprocity and trust					
	Gender segregation in play and friendships					
	Importance of large groups, clubs or gangs					
	Peer approval gains importance					
	Sees the importance of rules and wants to conform to them					

Table 1.3 An approximate guide to development in children: Key Stages 3 and 4 – 11–18 years old

| Physical attributes | Girls | Weight | 25–78 kg | Height | 130–175 cm | There are wide ranges and rapid growth spurts take place |
| | Boys | | 23–90 kg | | 130–191 cm | |

Move to biological maturity

Commencement of puberty with secondary sex characteristic development and the maturation of sexual organs

Development of body odour and possibly acne

Sleep patterns change

Girls

Commencement of puberty 8½–12½ years of age

Oestrogen stimulates growth and development of reproductive organs

Breast development

Growth of pubic and axillary hair

Rapid growth in height

First menstruation approximately 2½ years after start of puberty

Boys

Commencement of puberty 10–14½ years of age

Androgens, largely testosterone, stimulate growth and development of the reproductive organs

Testicular enlargement and growth in length and girth of penis

Change in voice with lowering of pitch of voice

Growth in height later and more marked than in girls

Hair growth in pubic, axillary face and chest areas

Gross motor	Achieving adult skills and strengths but activity often decreasing, particularly for girls
Fine motor	More skilled in areas of choice
Cognitive	Able to think in abstract terms
	Hold strong beliefs
	Sees others' points of view
Social emotional and behavioural	Mood swings in evidence possibly as result of hormones or of different and changing expectations
	Confidence develops and becoming more independent
	Developing own identity separate from family
	Friendship based on intimacy

need to consider factors that might impact upon children to make these differences in their physical growth and development evident. Some, but by no means all, potential factors are considered below.

Hereditary

Do we turn out like our parents? Clearly there is a genetic influence in some areas, as illustrated in a condition such as cystic fibrosis, a chronic illness from autosomal recessive inheritance when the individual inherits the defective gene from both parents. Being colour blind is genetically determined, with the genetic variant only carried on the X chromosome with a woman as the carrier. Other factors are genetic, or perhaps familiar, as the links may not have been explored, are not as clear cut, or there is a huge gene pool to consider. Height, academic ability and even the age at which children become dry at night seem to have a familiar or genetic element, but in everyday practice they are not easy to establish. This is compounded by the impact of so many factors: nutrition, early years stimulation and bedtime routine might interact with the three examples respectively cited above. The examination of these and other factors has led to the ongoing debate as to whether nature or nurture is responsible.

Gender differences

Discussion of gender can lead to a sharing of stereotypes, reinforcing traditional views that girls are more nurturing and boys more aggressive, as well

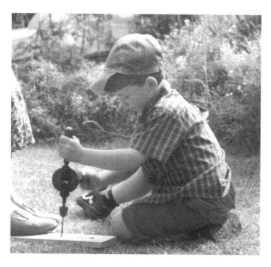

Children develop sophisticated fine motor skills.

as querying the assumption that boys cannot knit and girls do not want to play football. The actual situation is more difficult to establish. Boys are generally taller than girls when fully grown, but girls are currently doing better at school. In 2005, 62.1% of girls achieved five or more GCSEs at A*–C, compared with 52.2% of boys (DfES, 2006). In 1999 boys were more likely to have a mental disorder than girls and this was evident in both the 5–10 year age group and the 11–15 year age group. More specifically, the prevalence of conduct and hyperkinetic disorders were greater among boys than girls (Meltzer *et al.*, 2000). In 2000 there were higher proportions of boys rather than girls with both mild and severe disabilities (ONS, 2004). Can it be argued that these differences are directly from gender? Certainly some studies have indicated that the brains of males and females are distinct and work in a different way (Haier *et al.*, 2005). Educational achievement might be from styles of teaching assessment and expectation of both boys and girls. Mental health difficulties also could be influenced by up-bringing, styles of parenting and socialisation. Physical disabilities could have a biological basis, but even then the causes of disability need to be examined. Do some disabilities originate from risk-taking behaviour, which perhaps is more encouraged or likely in boys? We can say that height, body shape and sexual characteristics have biological, genetic and hormonal origins. Saying that other outcomes are a result of gender is more difficult.

Nutrition

There would be no disagreement that insufficient food in childhood is undesirable and affects the child's growth and development. The majority of children in the Western world have sufficient food but may well suffer from malnutrition or sub-nutrition, getting inadequate amounts of some nutrients and too much of foods that lead to obesity.

Children need a healthy and varied diet to help reduce the risk of heart disease, stroke, diabetes and osteoporosis in the future. It is also vital to contribute to their sense of well-being now, to sustain good mental health and promote healthy development. This diet should be built around carbohydrates, with protein and five or more portions of fruit and vegetables a day, as well as some fat and a low amount of salty and sugary food.

While many claim they know what they should be eating, the issue of obesity has been high on the agenda in recent years and the number of obese children has risen. The Health Survey for England (Joint Health Surveys Unit on behalf of the Department of Health, 2002) found that 8.5% of 6-year-olds and 15% of 15-year-olds were obese, with others being just overweight). Jeffery *et al.* (2005) surveyed and weighed parents and children and concluded that being overweight goes largely unrecognised; parents were poor at identifying being overweight in themselves and their children, and less likely to note it in their sons, revisiting the issue of gender. Obese children are less likely to take physical exercise. This is something that has declined in many children, yet as well as its health benefits physical exercise further develops gross motor skills.

Specific nutrient deficiencies will effect the child's development. A good supply of calcium, iron and vitamins A and D is necessary. Calcium is required for tooth development and, with vitamin D, helps make bones stronger. Iron deficiency anaemia is associated with frequent infections, poor weight gain and delay in development. Iron is most available in liver and red meat which is not always well received by children but can be offered as dark green leafy vegetables, pulses and nuts and in some fortified breakfast cereals. Taking in vitamin C through fruit or orange juice with a meal can increase the uptake of iron. Improving nutrition to support growth and development involves knowing what to eat and being willing and able to do so. Issues of health promotion will be considered in Chapter 2, but children may well be influenced by their psychological development, what the rest of the peer group will eat, if the food is available and if they or their parents can afford it.

Emotional well-being – relationships

If a key question is whether nature or nurture defines the child's growth and development, consideration of their mental well-being and the relationships each child has with parents, siblings and other children takes the investigation further into the nurture arena.

Much has been written about attachment, based on the work of Bowlby (1983) and his followers. Attachment is concerned with the relationship between two people, usually, though not always, mother and baby. Debates about the timing of attachment, and with whom, are many, but not all attachments are the same and Ainsworth *et al.* (1978) categorised attachment as secure; anxious–avoidant; and insecure–ambivalent with only the secure attachment having a two way responsive relationship between mother and baby. Considering the orbitofrontal part of the brain which is concerned with social responses, Gerhardt (2004) argued that development is experience-dependent, influenced by the child's interactions and relationships with people. Romanian orphans who had been severely neglected within orphanages had a virtual black hole in their orbitofrontal cortex which was related to emotions and the later forming of relationships (Chugani *et al.*, 2001). The quality of the early relationship has an impact on the child's later relationships. Securely attached babies are likely to become more confident, socially orientated, cooperative, and outgoing, and to have more friends (La Freniere and Sroufe, 1985).

Many writers have considered that it all hinges on the early weeks of the child's life, but those dealing with school-aged children might be more concerned with the significant ongoing relationships. Children whose self-esteem is challenged by a lack of encouragement, or even acknowledgement, from those around them may well not progress as expected. Individuals coping with disrupted relationships and persistent negative feedback may become withdrawn and isolated, lacking in motivation and reluctant to join in with others and use their developing skills, whether they are reading, swimming or something else.

Opportunity to practice

Reading through Tables 1.1 and 1.2 one could quite rightly say that a child will not learn to ride a two-wheeler bike if she does not have one, and learning to play a clarinet requires access to the instrument. The same can be applied to cognitive development. The child with limited conversational opportunities with adults is likely to have a less developed vocabulary. If she has little experience of books and does not see them used or valued this may impact on her enthusiasm and commitment to reading. The reasons why a child might receive little conversational stimulation or access to a bicycle may be very different, ranging from parental depression, poor parent–child relationship, lack of understanding of the need to interact with the child, stress and worry, socioeconomic restrictions and more.

Consideration of these and other factors impacting on a child's physical development highlights the interaction and complexity of the issues. The child's development is by no means predetermined. The role of relationships and the opportunity to practice point the reader towards psychological and social factors; these, with biological concerns, inter-link, making the headings of physical, psychological and social purely arbitrary.

Psychological

In considering psychological and cognitive development, there are different theoretical approaches that help organise and make sense of the vast amounts of information available. Some of the best known approaches have drawn on the work of Skinner, Piaget, Vygotsky and Bronfenbrenner (further detail on the work of these developmental psychologists is available in any quality child development text, such as Bee and Boyd (2007) or Berk (2006).

Psychologists can be seen to take a nativist, empiricist or constructivist approach (Woods, 2005). Over-simplistically, it can be said that nativists see the child as genetically pre-programmed, with the environment having little impact on the child's development, while the empiricists view the child as a blank slate, with children passive in their learning and ready to be shaped by parents and those around them. Constructivism acknowledges that the child has cognitive potential and views the child's development as a combination of the pre-programming and environmental adaptation. Empiricists veer towards the work of behaviourists, such as Pavlov, who described classical conditioning with dogs, and Skinner, who talked of operant conditioning, in his case with rats. Taking these two different approaches the child might receive a negative response or punishment for an undesirable behaviour and would be praised for doing something desirable in the hope that the positive behaviour is repeated in the future. Before we dismiss these views of child management, it is worth thinking about 'being kept in at playtime', using a star chart to encourage night time continence or stickers being handed out for participating well in a group activity, all approaches well used by parents and teachers.

The constructivist approach has been dominant in school-based education and in health education or promotion by health workers. Seeing the importance of the child's relationship with the environment draws heavily on the work of Piaget and Vygotsky.

For Piaget the child was a self-motivated explorer, constantly interacting with his physical world, realising the shortcomings of his way of thinking and revisiting it to modify it in line with his external reality. This was done by developing and adapting schema or categories, by experiencing his world and comparing it to his other experiences. Different information was then assimilated and absorbed into the schema. The child may have a clear idea of category of horse: a large creature, with four legs that is seen in fields. On seeing a camel for the first time, it may be assimilated into this category, but on observation of the humps, or an adult pointing out the differences in its appearance or eating habits, the child may come to see that it can no longer be assimilated into the schema as a 'lumpy horse'. The existing schema may then need accommodation, as it is adjusted, or a new schema created, of zoo animals or of camels, that gives a better fit. Throughout, the child is striving for coherence and seeking equilibrium; his understanding of the world is held in balance by constant changes in his schema.

The example of the lumpy camel shows the importance of language, which was also significant in Vygotsky's thinking. However, Piaget saw language as an outward sign of what was taking place while Vygostsky sees language as part of the process of cognitive development.

Piaget's cognitive–developmental stage theory had four stages: sensorimotor, preoperational, concrete operational, and formal operational. During the sensorimotor stage, from birth to about the age of two years of age, children are finding out how to learn. The major tasks occurring during this period involve children working out how to make use of their bodies. They do this by

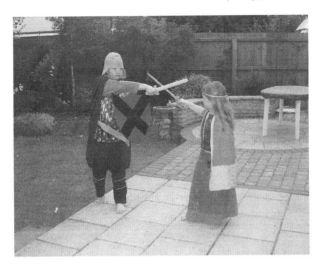

Imaginative play is important and fun for children.

experiencing everything with their five senses, and by learning to crawl and then walk, point and then grasp.

During the preoperational stage, roughly from ages two to seven, children start to use symbols or representations to understand and to interact with the world, and they begin to learn language and to engage in pretend play. They do not have clear rules that they apply to the world as they are working in a wide schema. Their thinking is rigid and they can only see one aspect of a situation, invariably their own. They may see inanimate objects as living and they have an inability to 'conserve'. They do not realise that physical characteristics stay the same when outward characteristics change, as shown in Piaget's classic experiment with the same amount of fluid in different shaped containers. In the concrete operational stage, lasting from approximately the ages of seven to eleven, children gain the ability to think logically, to solve problems and to organise information they learn. A nine-year-old may have categorised the different home and away kits of all the football teams in the Premier League. Information can be ranked and children may be able to have a clear view of who has the biggest and smallest shoe size in a class of 29 children. While their abilities may appear great, they remain limited to considering only concrete, not abstract, information. Finally, during the formal operational stage, which often lasts from age eleven on (and we might consider whether some ever reach it), adolescents learn how to think more abstractly, to solve problems and to think symbolically; that is, about things that are not concretely in front of them.

Piaget has been criticised; it has been suggested that he underestimated the capabilities of the child and that context and the environment can make quite a difference to what a child can do. While there are variations, a Piagetian approach puts the onus on the child; he develops in isolation, testing his theories as he makes an understanding of his world.

Vygotsky, in comparison, saw the child as a social being from the start, with his learning and development embedded within his social relationships and language being central. Vygotsky viewed cognitive development as a product of a two-way process, where the child learned through shared problem solving experiences with parents, teachers, siblings or friends. To begin with the person interacting with the child takes most of the responsibility for leading the activity, but gradually the child directs what should be done. Vygotsky stressed the role of language, with adults using speech to transmit to children the body of knowledge in the area being considered. Children use their own internal speech to direct their behaviour, in the same way that the adults' speech had previously directed them; we may be aware of this speech not being internal, as the child gives a running commentary on what they are doing.

A key issue in Vygotsky´s theory is the idea that cognitive development is limited to a certain time area, called the 'zone of proximal development' (ZPD). The ZPD refers to the gap between what children can achieve alone and what they can achieve through problem solving under adult guidance or by working with more capable peers. The ZPD will change as the child becomes more skilled in the area in question. Bruner formalised many of Vygotsky's ideas into educational strategies, as shown in the idea of 'scaffolding' (Bruner, 1975), which describes the changing quality of support between adult and a child. The term was used to explore the type of aid provided by an adult for children learning how to carry out a task they could not perform alone. The concepts of scaffolding and the ZPD fit well together and can be a useful underpinning to education work with children, whether it is assisted discovery, active learning or children involved in 'plan, do and review'.

For Vygotsky, language had a central role in learning and development; by acquiring language, the child was provided with a means of thinking in new ways. Language was used by children to solve problems and to rehearse a solution before trying it out. However, for the child the main purpose of language is social: through it they can obtain help from others and thus solve problems. There are major differences between the approaches taken by those who follow Piaget and Vygotsky, which can be explored elsewhere, but both saw children as active learners, engaged in their environment and with language in evidence though playing a different role.

Bronfenbrenner (1979) can be seen as taking a yet wider view, moving from constructivism to social constructivism and seeing the child as a social actor. Using a bio-ecological approach he brought different aspects of the child's world together and considered how environmental factors mesh with the child's biological and psychological makeup, with the different parts interacting. Bronfenbrenner saw the child's world in concentric circles nested within each other. The microsystem related to the child's personal experience in his immediate environments. For the school-aged child this might include family, school, after-school club, peer group, brownie pack, gang, church group or Koran classes. The mesosystem was concerned with connections between microsystems; these might be informal and formal links, such as parent–teacher communication, sport or religious networks. The exosystem was concerned with environmental settings which only indirectly affect the child and his development, such as the parent's workplace or the family's economic position. Lastly the macrosystem was concerned with the larger cultural context, which might include the local and national economies, political culture and the ethnic culture related to that child. For Bronfenbenner each system contained roles, norms and rules that can powerfully shape development. We are all in a position to think of many other factors that interact with the child, and to debate the interaction between the different systems. Factors such as economic status may have an impact at every level.

Bronfenbrenner's work in human ecology has contributed to the view that all elements from family to economic and political structures can impact on the life course throughout childhood and beyond, but it remains difficult to see the extent of the impact of each constituent.

Social

Many have attempted to produce a systematic study of the physical and psychological development of the child. Psychologists have set out to map the behavioural, emotional, social and cognitive development of children, and indeed human beings, across the lifespan. Recently there has been an increasing awareness of the roles that culture and context play, in terms of both process and outcome. Definitions of the child or childhood are usually influenced by historical factors: cultural, ideological, economic and religious views. The wider community system is seen to, and does, impact on the child as does the child's immediate surroundings, all considered in Bronfenbrenner's ecological system above. Taking this approach, childhood rather than the child is socially constructed. It is a product of the discourses, the myths, accounts and views of children that abound in any time or culture (Wryness, 2006). What then is a child or childhood? Rather than looking for a particular definition there will be multiple realities (Stainton-Rogers, 1989).

These different views of children and childhood have been encapsulated as the child as a physical entity (our starting point), developmentally *en route* to adulthood (the view of developmental psychologists), evil, innocent, passive, vulnerable, having rights, and no doubt more.

Children have been regarded in various ways at different times in history but we are inevitably reliant on the material left behind and we may question its reliability.

Aries (1962), although questioned on his historical accuracy and interpretation of material using contemporary ideas, argued that there was no concept of childhood prior to the 15th century, but from then on they were portrayed in paintings or documents as different, rather than just as small adults. A 20th century view of earlier times was that there was little emotional involvement with the child until survival, which was by no means routine, was assured. This was supported by Montaigne's 16th century remark 'I have lost two or three children, not without regret but without great sorrow'. Pollack (1987) however, argued that parents have always showed a range of emotions to their children and that the loss of a child left some parents distraught with grief (Pollack, 1983).

The 17th and 18th centuries marked a time of great economic, religious and political change and there is evidence of diverse and changing constructions of the child. Calvinistic or puritan views portrayed the child as inherently sinful, requiring firm discipline. Views in the period of the Enlightenment portrayed the child as innocent and dependent, needing protection and guidance. Locke (1689) saw the child as an empty slate, ready to be taught or moulded and Rousseau, writing in the 18th century (accessible in a 1979 translation), viewed children as noble savages, inherently good. Either marked the child as very different from the adult and in need of help and guidance.

In the 19th century the dominant view of the child was as something that needed to be controlled, with the lives of young people in Britain constrained by organisational links whether through family, education or work (Spence, 2005). Children might be seen as separate or different from adults, but as children there were constraints on the age at which they could commence work in the mines or factories and the hours they could toil. From 1870 there was a compulsion to go to school until the age of 13. 'Child' might have become a construct, but there was little concept of 'youth'. Young people were frequently out at work but still very much under the control of parents, with no luxury of the time for preparation for adulthood (Spence, 2005). Thinking in the 20th century was rationalist, with the idea of individual children going through stages much as presented early in this chapter and evident in the writings of Piaget (Bee and Boyd, 2007). Families became smaller and were more child-centred, as was primary education following the Plowden report of 1967 (Central Advisory Council for Education England). Health and welfare services were formalised, with an increased emphasis on protection and the mantra of services for the child, following the Children Act 1989, was: 'the welfare of the child is paramount'.

This reflects a growing view that children have rights. The United Nations Declaration on the Rights of the Child 1985 stated they should be protected against exploitation and discrimination. The United Nations Convention on the Rights of the Child 1989 was a benchmark in rethinking about children and childhood (Alderton, 2005) as it stated they had rights to provision, protection and participation. Provision included care for well-being, education, health, rest and leisure. Protection rights were against physical and mental violence, neglect and discrimination. Participation rights incorporated a right to life, a name identity and nationality, a right to express views on matters that affected the child, freedom of expression and the right of a disabled child to enjoy a full and decent life.

At the end of the 20th century and beginning of the 21st children have been seen as both innocent in need of care and protection and as 'devils' in need of strict discipline. The James Bulger case, which has entered folk memory, represents these two views. In February 1993 a two-year-old, James Bulger, was taken from a shopping centre and murdered in a railway siding by ten-year-old boys. The murdered child was presented as vulnerable, as have older children who have been murder victims, irrespective of the perpetrator. The two boys who had committed the murder were seen as in need of discipline and incarceration, beliefs that have followed them into their adulthood. Goldson (2001) argues that we hold these two concepts of childhood in tandem. Children are seen as innocent and vulnerable, but when they move beyond the limits of what is seen as acceptable they are classified as different – a threat or a problem.

For others, children are seen something in which to invest, at both individual and collective levels. For the individual child this might be in the form of school fees or extra tuition to get the best from their education, or it could be extra sports coaching or presents or experiences from a family who never had these opportunities themselves. At community or societal level it again might be education, with an investment in schools, academies, or children's centres. With these and other inputs they will grow into the effective workers of the future, well endowed with education and skills to enhance the economy and ready to support their parents or (by tax) other older people in the community. Perhaps cynically the child can be seen as a product of effective, targeted health promotion, health care and education, the process monitored by bodies such as Ofsted and the Healthcare Commission.

The construction of children and childhood in the 21st century may be varied and so is the experience of individual children. Some will have responsive and consistent carers who provide good nutrition and quality education; others will grow up in unsupported and disrupted families and be subjected to bullying at school or in their neighbourhood.

Robb (2001) suggests that the changing experience of childhood can be considered under four headings: material circumstances; health; education; and play and leisure.

There is a belief that material circumstances have improved in the past thirty years, yet while some have regular foreign holidays and access to the latest technology, child poverty still exists. Figures released in 2007 showed that in 2005–6 3.8 million children in Britain were in poverty, in homes with less than 60% of average income including housing costs. Such households were more likely to be headed by a lone parent or by someone from an ethnic minority. Such families were often larger than the norm, having no one in work (perhaps because of a disability), and many such households were in inner London (Department of Work and Pensions [DWP], 2007). With televisions and DVDs commonly available they potentially increase the awareness of material resources to which some do not have access, therefore potentially increasing dissatisfaction. A UNICEF report in 2007, which collected indicators of child well-being in rich countries, concluded that children in the United Kingdom did less well than in the other 21 countries it considered (UNICEF Innocenti Research Centre, 2007).

There is confidence that health has improved and while epidemics are rare and life expectancy has increased there has been a growth in childhood obesity, with its implications for long-term health; and there is concern about the mental health of young people. Education has widened the age span with which it is concerned but many feel there is increased pressure on children to achieve and meet schools' targets, causing extra stress for the children and young people and often generating concern for parents. The increasing numbers staying in further or higher education have meant that young people are financially dependent on others, often their families, for a longer period than previous generations, while the reality of large debts from going into higher education was not an experience of the majority in the past.

If earlier puberty together with a prolonged time of financial dependence is a tension, so is the increased emphasis on leisure but with reduced independent mobility. A work–life balance is seen as important for all and exercise may offset the problems of obesity, but the majority of children and young people have their local movements constrained, perhaps for good reasons. A survey commissioned by Play England for Playday (2007) showed that 71% of adults played outside in the street or area close to their homes every day when they were children, compared with only 21% of children today.

These and other changes in the experience of childhood are not difficult to identify, but as Robb (2001) notes there has not been a straightforward linear change in children's experience. Perhaps reacting to an empiricist view, he reflects that children themselves are not passive, but social actors who at times shape their circumstances; those who have experience of children and young people may have clear ideas how.

Conclusion

This chapter has sought to show that children can and have been viewed in different ways. Dividing the viewpoints into physical, psychological and social is simplistic – the perspectives overlap and each is changing. With different and varying views of the child and childhood, we may in the 21st century have different perceptions of what makes a makes a happy, well-balanced child or young person. The starting point for the chapter was 'What are children and young people like?'. The answer might be 'What do you want them to be like?', and this is addressed by the models and framework that are used to construct the child and their childhood.

Bill Stone, a social worker linked with the National Society for the Prevention of Cruelty to Children and the Churches' Child Protection Advisory Service talked of the vision of childhood in the 21st century. For him it is characterised by a freedom to learn and grow, where the child can take for granted unconditional love and where the child experiences wonder, excitement and fulfilment. For Stone, good parenting and community links are part of achieving this. His vision of childhood may be different from that of the past and of some other cultures and even our own, but it is starting point with which many will agree.

References

Alderton, P. (2005) Children's rights. In: *Understanding Early Childhood. Issues and Controversies* (ed. H. Penn). Open University Press, Berkshire.

Aries, P. (1962) *The Centuries of Childhood*. Cape, London.

Ainsworth, M. D., Blehar, M. C., Waters, E. and Wall, S. (1978) *Patterns of Attachment: a Psychological Study of the Strange Situation*. Erlbaum, Hillsdale, NJ.

Bee, H. and Boyd, D. (2007) *The Developing Child*, 11th edn. Pearson Educational, Boston.

Berk, L. (2006) *Child Development*, 7th edn. Pearson, London.

Bowlby, J. (1953) *Child Care and the Growth of Love*. Penguin, Harmondsworth.

Bronfenbrenner, U. (1979) *The Ecology of Human Development*. Harvard University Press, Cambridge, MA.

Bruner, J. S. (1975) The ontogenesis of speech acts. *Journal of Child Language*, **2**, 1–40.

Central Advisory Council for Education (England) (1967) *Children and their Primary Schools. (The Plowden Report)*. HMSO, London.

Chugani, H., Behen, H., Muzik, O., Juhasz, C., Nagy, F. and Chungani, D. (2001) Local brain functional activity following early deprivation; a study of post-institutionalised Roumanian orphans. *Neuroimage*, **14**, 1290–310.

Department for Children, Schools and Families (2007) *Raising Expectations: Staying in Education and Training Post-16*. DCSF, London. http://www.dfes.gov.uk/publications/raisingexpectations; accessed 17 August 2007.

Department for Education and Skills (2006) *Education and Skills Find Out More. Gender and Achievement in Schools*. http://findoutmore.dfes.gov.uk/2006/07/gender_and_achi.html; accessed 1 October 2007.

Department for Education and Skills (2007) *Early Years Foundation Stage: Statutory Framework and Guidance*. DfES, London.

Department for Work and Pensions (2007) *Households Below Average Income (HBAI) 1994/95–2005/06* (Revised). http://www.dwp.gov.uk/asd/hbai/hbai2006/contents.asp; accessed 12 December 2007.

Gerhardt, S. (2004) *Why Love Matters. How Affection Shapes A Baby's Brain*. Brunner–Routledge, Hove.

Goldson, B. (2001) The demonisation of children: from the symbolic to the institutional. In: *Children in Society. Contemporary, Policy and Practice* (eds. P. Foley, J. Roche and S. Tucker). Palgrave, Basingstoke.

Haier, R. J., Jung, R. E., Yeo, R. A., Head, K. and Alkire, M. T. (2005) The neuroanatomy of general intelligence: sex matters. *Neuroimage*, **25**(1), 320–7.

Jeffery, A. N., Voss, L. D., Metcalf, B. S., Alba, S. and Wilkin, T. J. (2005) Parents' awareness of overweight in themselves and their children: cross-sectional study within a cohort (EarlyBird 21). *British Medical Journal*, **330**, 23–4.

Joint Health Surveys Unit on behalf of the Department of Health (2002) *Health Survey for England 2001*. Stationery Office, London.

La Freniere, P. and Sroufe, L. A. (1985) Profiles of peer competence in the pre-school: interrelations between measures, influence of social ecology, and relation to attachment history. *Developmental Psychology*, **21**, 56–9.

Locke, J. (1689) *An Essay Concerning Human Understanding*. http://books.google.co.uk/books; accessed 12 December 2007.

Meltzer, H., Gatwood, R., Goodman, R. and Ford, T. (2000) *Mental Health of Children and Adolescents in Great Britain*. Stationery Office, London.

Office for National Statistics (2002) *Young People in Education or Training: by Gender and Age, 1986 to 1999: Social Trends 31*. http://www.statistics.gov.uk/STATBASE/ssdataset.asp?vlnk=3433&More; accessed 17 August 2007.

Office of National Statistics (2004) *Disability: More Boys than Girls with Disability*. http://www.statistics.gov.uk/CCI/nugget.asp?ID=795&Pos=2&ColRank=2&Rank=864; accessed 17 August 2007.

Office of the High Commission for Human Rights (undated) The Convention on the Rights of the Child, adopted by the General Assembly of the United Nations in 1989. http://www.unhchr.ch/html/menu3/b/k2crc.htm. Accessed 14 December 2007.

Playday (2007) An ICM opinion poll on street play http://www.playday.org.uk/playday_campaigns/2007_our_streets_too/research.asp; accessed 1 October 2007.

Pollack, L. (1983) *Forgotten Children*. Cambridge University Press, Cambridge.

Pollack, L. (1987) *Parents and Children over Three Centuries*. Fourth Estate, London.

Robb, M. (2001) The changing experience of childhood. In: *Children in Society. Contemporary, Policy and Practice* (eds. P. Foley, J. Roche and S. Tucker). Palgrave, Basingstoke.

Rousseau, J. (1979) *Emile* (transl. Allan Bloom). Basic Books, New York.

Spence, J. (2005) Concepts of youth. In: *Working with Young People* (eds. R. Harrison and C. Wise). Sage/Open University, London.

Stainton-Rogers, R. (1989) The social construction of childhood. In: *Child Abuse and Neglect* (W. Stainton-Rogers, D. Harvey and E. Ash). Open University Press, London.

Stainton-Rogers, W. (2001) Constructing childhood, constructing child concern. In: *Children in Society. Contemporary, Policy and Practice* (eds. P. Foley, J. Roche and S. Tucker). Palgrave, Basingstoke.

Stone, B. (2007) A vision of childhood in the 21st century. *Caring Magazine*, Spring, 5–7.

UNICEF Innocenti Research Centre (2007). *Child Poverty in Perspective: an Overview of Child Well-being in Rich Countries*. Innocenti Research Centre, Florence.

Woods, M. (2005) Early childhood studies: first principles. In: *Early Childhood Studies. An Holistic Introduction*, 2nd edn (eds. J. Taylor and M. Woods). Hodder Arnold, London.

Wryness, M. (2006) *Childhood and Society. An Introduction to the Sociology of Childhood*. Palgrave Macmillan, Basingstoke.

Further reading

Bee, H. and Boyd, D. (2007) *The Developing Child*, 11th edn. Pearson Educational, Boston.

Berk, L. (2006) *Child Development*, 7th edn. Pearson, London.

Drennan, V. and Goodman, C. (eds.) (2007) *Oxford Handbook of Primary Care and Community Nursing*. Oxford University Press, Oxford.

Glasper, A., McEwing, G. and Richardson, J. (eds.) (2007) *Oxford Handbook of Children's and Young People's Nursing*. Oxford University Press, Oxford.

James, A. and James, A. (2004) *Constructing Childhood: Theory, Policy, and Social Practice*: Palgrave Macmillan, Basingstoke.

Useful website

Enuresis Resource and Information Centre (ERIC): http://www.ERIC.org.UK/.

CHAPTER 2

Promoting health: historical overview and political context

Sarah Sherwin and Alison Williams

Key themes

- The historical perspective of policy and legislation affecting services for school-age children and young people.
- The integration of health, education and social care.
- An overview of the development of school health services.

Introduction

Promoting the health of school-aged children has traditionally focused on providing them with information about how to live a healthy lifestyle and reduce risk-taking behaviours to protect their future health. Decisions made today by children, young people and their parents in the United Kingdom (UK) are affecting their health now, in childhood, into adulthood, and beyond. Childhood obesity is increasing year on year (Department of Health [DH], 2004a), teenage pregnancies are the highest in Europe (Health Development Agency, 2004), sexually transmitted infections are prevalent amongst those under 25 years (Health Protection Agency, 2005), and the UK has one of the highest levels of binge drinking in Europe amongst teenagers (Alcohol Concern, 2007). A significant number of 11–15 year olds are regularly smoking (NHS Health and Social Care Information Centre, 2006), and many young people struggle with low self-esteem and the number who self harm is estimated to be 1:15 (Mental Health Foundation, 2007). The need to protect and safeguard children and young people has also risen to a new level in recent years (Laming, 2003). Young adults who have not done well in school are more at risk of living in poverty, being involved in crime and having health problems (DfES, 2006a).

All of these issues pose serious public health challenges, as the personal, economic and societal costs are huge. There needs to be a better awareness and understanding of the underlying causes that affect health and health behaviours in order to instigate change. In order to respond to these public health issues there has been a plethora of reports, policies and guidance documents produced to support the promotion and protection of the health of today's children and young people. This chapter aims to explore the key drivers for change and the historical background to these changes.

Policy affecting children's health services

The Laming Report (2003) highlighted the extent of fragmentation between services and the need to improve joint working and better communication. Children's Trusts were created to address such issues by formalising joint working and maximising resources. This is underpinned by the duty to cooperate in the *Children Act* (DH, 2004b), the *National Service Framework for Children, Young People and Maternity Services* (DH, 2004c), *Every Child Matters* (DH/DfES, 2004) and *Youth Matters* (DfES, 2005a). This children's agenda is a national programme of system-wide reform specifically designed to ensure that all children's services are working together alongside parents and carers to provide increased opportunities for children and young people.

Government initiatives and policies (DH, 1999b; DH, 2004c) have reinforced the belief that promoting health should be the responsibility of every practitioner. *Every Child Matters* (DH/DfES, 2004) and *Youth Matters* (DfES, 2005a) have influenced how schools and other services work with children and young people up to the age of 19 (and 25 for those with learning disabilities). They promote health, both physical and emotional, as well as providing guidance on safeguarding children and young people. *Every Child Matters* was given legal status in the form of the *Children Act* (DH, 2004b) and makes it clear that it is everyone's responsibility to help achieve the five key outcomes outlined. Achieving these outcomes can only occur if there is more joined up thinking between agencies, both statutory and voluntary. Consultation and engagement with young people also need to feature heavily in the development and delivery of services.

Overview of the development of the school health service

The school health service began to develop in the late 19th century, when a medical officer for schools was first appointed in London in 1890. This was followed two years later by the employment of the first school nurse. In 1882 a policy issued by the Department of Education stated that school managers could close schools or exclude pupils from attending in order to control the spread of infectious diseases (Harris, 1995). This recognised that there was a relationship between health, the school environment and pupils reaching their full potential.

The Education (Administrative Provisions) Act of 1907 placed a legal obligation on schools to consider the health of the children in their care. It stated that it was the duty of school boards to provide for a medical inspection on admission to a public elementary school. This followed the recommendations from the Interdepartmental Committee on Physical Deterioration in 1904 that a national school health service should be established, staffed by qualified nurses and medical officers. These recommendations were made following concerns that approximately 60% of potential army recruits were deemed to be physically unfit for duty. The main reasons were poor eyesight, dental caries, heart disease and unsatisfactory growth, many of which had started during childhood (Leff and Leff, 1959). The publication of this report marked a turning point in the history of public health. Not only did it recommend the setting up a school health service, but it led the way for the introduction of a number of further public health reforms which would also impact on children's and young people's health.

Although there was a recognition that the status of children's health also impacted on other aspects of their lives, the focus of the early school health service was largely reactive. It concentrated on identifying physical health problems, detecting and treating poor hygiene and malnutrition and improving conditions for those with disability (Spencer, 1998). The Education Act of 1918 extended the duties of local education authorities requiring provision to be made for the treatment of minor ailments within primary schools, and medical inspections to be carried out for those in secondary education by school medical officers. Despite this reactive focus on the provision of treatment and issuing of advice, there was also an emphasis on the need to promote health linking the service back to its original public health roots (British Paediatric Association, 1995).

During the 1950s the role of the school nurse was largely concerned with screening, conducting hygiene inspections and providing advice relating to the control and treatment of infectious diseases, but there was concern relating to young people's emotional health and well-being. Leff and Leff (1959) describe how school nurses supported teenage girls in secondary schools, and today this supportive role, for both boys and girls, remains a key aspect of contemporary school nursing practice. The establishment of school nurse 'drop-in clinics' provides this type of support but interestingly is considered to be a relatively new development of service provision.

In 1974 the school health service transferred from the control of Local Authorities to the National Health Service. This was a major event for school health staff as it meant a change of employer. Although this caused dilemmas for some, a more positive effect was that nurses became more politically aware: it strengthened professional unity and provided more opportunities for professional development (Strehlow, 1987).

Under the reorganisation it was recommended that Local Education Authorities and Area Health Authorities worked collaboratively to promote the interests of children. One of the aims of this 'new health service for children' was to provide an integrated health service bringing together different health professionals such as community and hospital paediatricians, clinical medical officers, school nurses, audiologists, speech and language therapists, psychologists and community physiotherapists. This approach stemmed back to 1907 when the Board of Education stated that the medical services for children should be unified and delivered based on the needs of the communities they served. This indicates that the service had its roots firmly planted within the philosophy of public health, albeit based within a particular school environment.

The Court Report (Court Committee Report, 1976) recommended that all children should receive a detailed medical examination on entering school by a school doctor and have an annual interview with a school nurse. Consultant paediatricians were appointed to provide leadership to the school medical officers. The report was generally considered to be impractical by the education authorities as the recommendations centred largely on the interests of doctors rather than educationalists (Johnson, 1977). However, there were significant recommendations relating to training for school nurses, which were in part implemented.

The 1981 Education Act related to both health and education services. It required health authorities to notify education authorities about children with a disability or special educational needs. This will be discussed further in Chapter 10.

The Children Act (DH, 1989) provided a legal framework encouraging health, education and social services to work together more closely in identifying children in need such as those with disabilities as well as those requiring protection.

Government reforms such as the *Health of the Nation* (DH, 1992) required health professionals to promote children's and young people's health and looked at the importance of assessing need in order to target services. *Saving Lives, Our Healthier Nation* (DH, 1999b) took a stronger public health approach and specifically discussed school nurses and the important strategic role they can play in promoting the health of school age children and young people.

School nurse training and professional development

By the end of 1955 there were over 6,000 school nurses working in England (Leff and Leff, 1959). A survey conducted by the Royal College of Nursing in 2005 (Ball and Pike, 2005) found that since the mid-1950s the number of school nurses had dropped significantly. There are now fewer than 3,000 school nurses (many of these working part-time) who are employed to cover the whole of the United Kingdom, and of these only 856 had a specialist school nurse qualification. Not surprisingly the school nursing service has often been described as being invisible, as much of the job is conducted outside of traditional NHS settings and based within schools. There has also been an assumption that there is little published research relating to school nursing practice. In 2006, Debell and Tomkins conducted a scoping exercise to clarify the evidence base for school nursing which disputed this view and identified that there is a considerable amount of evidence which supports school nursing practice.

A major landmark in school nurse professional development was the recommendation of specialist training by the Court Report in addition to their general nursing qualification. This helped to raise the profile of the service and enabled school nurses to function more effectively as the health representative within education (While and Barriball, 1993). In the late 1990s the training became a degree qualification which brought it in line with other community nurse post-registration training. School nurse education is now far more wide ranging than just delivering health care within school environments and practitioners have to meet standards of proficiency in public health nursing (see Table 2.1). The recognised education route leads to the qualification of a specialist community public health nurse with registration onto the third part of the Nursing and Midwifery Council Register (NMC, 2004), currently annotated as a school nurse.

One of the major criticisms of school health services over the last century has been the diversity of service delivery. In 2000 there was an attempt by DeBell and Jackson to bring together some of the differences across the country. They sug-

Table 2.1 Standards of proficiency for entry to Specialist Community Public Health Nursing NMC Register (NMC 2004).

- Surveillance and assessment of the population's health and well-being.
- Collaborative working for health and well-being.
- Working with, and for, communities to improve health and well-being.
- Developing health programmes and services and reducing inequalities.
- Policy and strategy development and implementation to improve health and well-being.
- Research and development to improve health and well-being.
- Promoting and protecting the population's health and well-being.
- Developing quality and risk management within an evaluative culture.
- Strategic leadership for health and well-being.
- Ethically managing self, people and resources to improve health and well-being.

gested a broad aim and service objectives that could be the focus for all school health services and identified a multi-skilled team structure incorporating a school nurse advisor, specialist practitioner team leader, community staff nurses and support workers. This was generally a new way of thinking as school nursing services had a flat structure with all of the nurses employed on the same pay grade doing the same roles. Although this strategy was not universally adopted initially it has paved the way for the recent developments within school nursing and encouraged different areas to review their own levels of service provision and introduce change. Many school nursing teams now have a structure comprising a team leader, specialist practitioners, staff nurses and support workers.

Recent health policies and guidance have recognised the contribution school nurses make in promoting health and identifying health needs (DH, 1999b; DH, 2004a,c,d; DH, 2006; DH/DfES, 2003). *Saving Lives: Our Healthier Nation* (DH, 1999b) suggested that school nurses should lead teams in order to identify, deliver and evaluate services for school age children and young people. *Health for All Children* (Hall and Elliman, 2003) challenged whether all children should be offered health screening and suggested that services should focus more on selective screening and surveillance. This would then allow school nursing services to extend their public health remit. Later, *Choosing Health: Making Healthier Choices Easier* (DH, 2004a) recommended that the number of qualified school nurse practitioners should increase significantly and that there should be a qualified school nurse public health practitioner for every cluster of primary schools and the related secondary school by 2010. With the introduction of practice-based commissioning and the merging of health, education and social care school nursing services need to work with key stakeholders in order to deliver, expand and develop appropriate provision that meet the needs of children and young people. Although employed by primary care trusts there are a number of models emerging where individual schools are purchasing school health services directly. *Looking for a School Nurse* (DH, 2006) is a guide aimed at head teachers and governors to help them work with school nursing services.

School nurses also have to respond to the wider public health agenda and consider how the health needs of the school age population are being met in both the state and independent sectors and outside the formal school environment. Public health is strengthened by sound needs assessment and this is addressed in Chapter 3.

The role of schools in promoting health

Schools can play a significant part in providing for children's and young people's personal, social and health education (PSHE) as well as creating opportunities for their spiritual, moral and cultural development (Office for Standards in Education [Ofsted], 2005). Schools are seen as an important setting for promoting health, reaching a large number of children and young people over a number of years from early childhood to adolescence (Naidoo and Wills, 2000). The purpose of health education within the curriculum is to provide children and young people with a working knowledge about issues that are important to their health (Spencer, 1998). However, what they do with the information depends on their personal priorities, their resources, their perception of risk to their long-term health and how much they value themselves. A report compiled by Ofsted (2005) supports the concept that health education is about providing information and knowledge, but argues that this alone is not sufficient. It is also important for children and young people to have the opportunity to formulate, develop and explore their own values and attitudes to health.

Despite acknowledgement that PSHE is a valuable and vital aspect of education it remains a non-statutory subject within the National Curriculum, so it can become marginalised within the curriculum (Naidoo and Wills, 2000).

Documents such as *Every Child Matters* (DH/DfES, 2004) and *National Healthy School Status: A Guide for Schools* (DfES, 2005b) highlight the responsibilities schools have to ensure that children and young people achieve better outcomes in relation to their health, which impacts on their learning.

PSHE is discussed in more detail in Chapter 5.

Whole school approach

The number of schools and the diversity of school settings within the UK is huge. The types and structure of schools vary between local authorities and may include primary/infant/junior schools, middle schools, secondary/high schools, special schools, specialist units, faith schools, specialist schools, trust schools and academies. In addition to state provision there are a host of independent schools. Schools vary enormously in size, ranging from rural schools with pupil numbers of 50 or below to large secondary schools with pupil numbers in excess of 1500. The range of curriculum topics, facilities and resources available to pupils as well as the specialist knowledge of staff employed to deliver and support learning is diverse. The identification and meeting of health needs in a range of different settings is challenging. Generally it is the head teacher, senior management team and governing body that are responsible for the type and content of the curriculum delivered in each school. Head teachers are often seen as gatekeepers to individual school communities and they generally control what takes place within the school. In some schools head teachers have not always considered health to be a priority and consequently it hasn't featured highly on schools' agendas. However, all schools are now being asked to consider the importance of physical health and emotional well-being and the part that these play in maximising the potential of children and their learning. The move towards adopting a more holistic whole school approach is a key change in thinking about the school environment. The introduction of the Healthy Schools Programme (DH, 1999a) and subsequent guidance (DfES, 2004a; 2005b) is an attempt to link government policies and programmes relating to health. A positive school environment can increase the sense of achievement and success, leading to greater feeling of well-being and satisfaction.

The whole school approach to health is not new: it was advocated back in 1939 when the Board of Education published a handbook *Suggestions on Health Education* (McNalty, 1939). However, it failed to make much impact within the education system. A whole school approach aims to bring about cultural changes within the school environment in relation to how health is viewed and promoted. A key aspect is the participation of the whole school community, including pupils, parents, governors, teachers, teaching assistants, site managers, and catering and cleaning staff, as well as others linked to the school such as school health personnel, Connexions advisors and representatives from the local community.

Although the Healthy Schools Programme was introduced back in 1999, not all schools engaged with the programme and in 2005 it was decided to take a more rigorous approach; all schools are now required to participate. To gain healthy schools status, schools have to demonstrate and provide evidence of how the programme is embedded into school life, including details of strategic planning outlined within the school improvement plan. Measuring the long-term effectiveness and impact of the healthy schools programme on children, young people and school communities is more challenging. In order to assess the impact of healthy schools a longitudinal evaluation study is being undertaken through the *Every Child Matters* agenda.

Specific health issues such as obesity can be highlighted through the healthy schools initiative and the Government is committed to tackling obesity through education in a number of ways. This includes improving food in schools with more healthy choices and improving the amount of exercise children undertake in and out of the school setting (DfES, 2005e). Ofsted also has a responsibility to monitor food standards and the challenge for schools and school caterers is to provide healthy food, which is presented and packaged in an acceptable way to persuade young people to buy it. There are increasing calls for young people to learn more about food and cooking healthy food as part of the curriculum. Although the science of food is part of the curriculum, cooking and shopping for appropriate food are not. In conjunction with this there is an effort through education and out of school activities to offer more attractive ways to encourage children and young people to take more exercise. All this will require engagement of parents in the process and needs a whole school approach to healthy food and exercise (DCSF, 2008).

Parents and carers have a vital and important part to play within the healthy schools agenda. However, a more collaborative approach between parents, schools, health services and others such as community workers, needs to exist to enable them to work together in a more holistic way, so that children and young people receive consistent messages relating to health issues. Parents and carers need to be more involved within the school's curriculum and to be active from the outset in health initiatives Their involvement would mean that health messages are underpinned and reinforced at home rather than just aiming the intervention at the pupils, who may have little control over their family's lifestyle. Parents can be involved through Parent Councils that are being established as part of the recommendations outlined in *Higher Standards Better Schools for All: More Choice for Parents and Pupils* (DfES, 2005c). *Parents Know How* (DCSF, 2007b) is another example of how support can be given to parents when they need it most. Information can be sent via instant messaging or text to help parents with their children on a variety of issues, such as how to reduce obesity and supporting children who have been bullied. This will help to ensure that the importance of adopting a healthy lifestyle is taught at school within the PSHE curriculum is underpinned by a whole school ethos toward health as advocated by the *Healthy Schools Programme* (DH, 1999a) and then key messages are further supported and reinforced by parents and carers at home.

Partnership working between health, education and social care

Working alongside other agencies has been a central feature of the school health service. However, it may be more accurate to describe this as parallel working rather than true partnership. There have been challenges over the years as school health services have only been able to work in schools by invitation. Often social workers, education staff and school health have all been working with a child and their family with often little communication taking place between the different agencies. *Every Child Matters* (DH/DfES, 2003), and the *Children Act* (DH, 2004b) seeks to address some of these shortcomings in the establishment of Children's Trust.

Every Child Matters: Changes for Children (DH/DfES, 2004) outlined plans to integrate children's services in a single organisation in the form of Children's Trusts. The aim of such Trusts is to involve children and their families in developing services designed around their needs. This should be achieved through public, private and voluntary and community providers (Davies, 2007). Children's Trusts will support the development of initiatives such as Extended Schools. There is no definitive 'blueprint' of what an extended school must look like as it should meet the needs of an individual community's and reflect its diversity (National Governors' Association [NGA], 2006).

The Government pledged that by 2010:

> 'All children should have access to a variety of activities beyond the school day' and that these will give them 'the opportunity to keep fit and healthy, to acquire new skills, to build on what they learn during the school day or simply to have fun and relax' (DfES, 2005c, p. 4).

Extended schools will be expected to provide a core offer including a variety of services and activities outside of school hours. The intention is to build a base for parental support, to have easy access to services and to develop communities (DfES, 2004b; 2005d; 2006b,c).

During 2006–08 funding has been invested to support schools in developing extended services. However, it is crucial that services developed are sustainable. The DfES (2006c) provided guidance on this for schools. Suggestions by the DCSF (2007a) as sources of funding include neighbourhood renewal, Learning and Skills Council and the Big Lottery Fund, PESSCL (physical education, school sport and club links) strategy funding and Working Tax Credit.

Fundamental to the development of extended services is the consultation and involvement of the wider community. The Education Act (2002) places a statutory requirement on school governing bodies to consult widely before providing extended services and to increase the range of those services by working in partnership with other service providers. The impact of extended schools on children's behaviour and engagement with learning has been recognised (DCSF, 2007a) and increased funding to support services enabling disadvantaged children to have free access to the activities has been committed (Wilkin *et al.*, 2003).

Extended services and health

Addressing health needs through extended schools offers potential benefits such as improving pupils' attendance, removing barriers to learning through earlier intervention, improving take up of preventative health services and reaching hard-to-access communities (DfES, 2006b). Schools that deliver services on site have found that children and young people and their parents feel more confident about accessing them (DfES, 2006c), benefit from travel and time costs and are more likely to keep appointments. From 2008 a number of support infrastructures will aid swift and easy referral core delivery including Children's Trusts, contact points for practitioners, use of the Common Assessment Framework, local area agreements and children's and young people's plans.

Although the local Children's Trust will be responsible for commissioning specialist services, schools will have a key role in influencing priorities and service design. Schools have a responsibility to ensure that all staff, especially support staff with pastoral, mentoring or family link roles, understand what services are available, criteria for referral and the best way to refer an individual. School nurses can act as a bridge between education, health and social care by supporting work on health issues and helping to make health services more accessible to children, young people, parents, carers and staff (DH, 2006).

Although most schools value the input of school health services, there can be conflict when the school nurse wishes to extend the boundaries of health care, such as by providing emergency contraception, issuing condoms and offering pregnancy testing within the school setting. School nurses play a pivotal role in identifying, meeting and evaluating the needs of children and young people, but it is vital that provision is not just a school health service but a service for school age children and young people (Madge and Franklin, 2003). The importance of collaboration and partnership working must continue to be one of the driving forces directing the development of services for children and young people (this is discussed further in Chapter 13). The evolvement of children trusts, children's centres and extended schools, bringing together health, social care and education, aims to provide and deliver accessible services at the heart of communities in order to deliver more holistic, integrated services (DH, 2004a).

Models of delivery

In many instances the identification of schools or clusters to develop extended services has taken into account current key developments already in existence such as Children's Centres. These centres already have a focus on multi-agency support for children and young people. The appropriate model of delivery will of course depend on the schools' existing resources and objectives. Such examples include direct delivery, delivering with a third party, linking with school clusters and co-locating with Children's Centres (DfES, 2006a). The underpinning principles of extended schools are closely aligned with the Healthy Schools Programme (DH, 1999a). Much of the work involved in meeting the criteria for healthy schools status assists schools in developing extended services. There are other developments within schools such as SEAL (social and emotional aspects of learning); new inspection framework and self-evaluation will support schools in developing the *Every Child Matters* agenda. Extended services, workforce reform and building diverse teams across agencies and at different levels are required to meet identified needs. School governors now have a duty to promote the well-being of pupils, community cohesion and safer schools partnerships (DCSF, 2007a).

Monitoring success

There is evidence that extended schools have led to improvements in attainment and engagement in learning, and have narrowed the achievement gap for the most disadvantaged children (DCSF, 2007a). Between 2005 and 2006 extended schools improved at twice the national average in both Key Stages 2 and 4. However, other less quantifiable predicted outcomes have been difficult to measure (see below).

Chamberlain *et al.* (2006) looked at potential advantages and disadvantages of extended schools taking the views of all stakeholders. Provision across primary and secondary schools was similar, with primary schools advocating that facilities should be used more for community access, such as breakfast clubs and secondary schools offering more opportunities for family learning. While the DfES (2005d) guidance outlined provision for all schools to be providing extended services by 2010, the survey showed that extended services were more evident in schools with the greatest need: schools with higher levels of free school meals, lower levels of attainment or higher percentage of pupils with English as an additional language. Pupils reported the main advantage being the wider range of extracurricular activities, with parents highlighting the primary advantage as increased supervision time for their children alongside the opportunity for 'one stop shops' for health and other services. Interestingly Chamberlain *et al.* (2006) reported that parents did not highlight any disadvantages. Conversely, staff felt there were few advantages, with less than 10% identifying improved behaviour or attainment. Concerns were also raised around increased workloads and longer hours.

The ultimate aim of extended services is to raise the standards and achievements of children and young people (Ofsted, 2006), but surveys and research to date have shown that the impact has been difficult to measure.

There is a risk of just considering easily quantifiable outcomes such as attainment and attendance. Perhaps focusing on the difference the service intends to make for children and young people may help to measure the baseline and outcomes so that services can be evaluated and resources used efficiently (DfES, 2006b).

Challenges

Integrated service delivery should be built on partnerships across services and does not just involve extended schools taking on these diverse roles or owning the agenda (DfES, 2006c). Whatever the model of delivery, the schools need to ensure that the staff (whether they are school staff, children's service staff, health partners, voluntary or private employees) are appropriately qualified and that safeguarding procedures have been rigorously followed (NGA, 2006). Within each local area there is an Extended Schools Adviser who has specific responsibility for supporting the development of extended schools and bringing together professionals from across all the agencies to plan effectively and sustain provision which meets local needs (DfES, 2005d). A key challenge is to address the school staff's concerns about workload. A culture shift is required if the Government's ideology for teachers and support staff to work with both current new partners is to be actualised (DfES, 2005d), rather than them being expected just to deliver extended activities.

There seem to be a number of key messages from early pilot sites that support the successful implementation of extended schools. These include the importance of early consultations with key groups, establishing contracts and formal agreements, understanding roles and responsibilities and training the workforce (DfES, 2005d).

Agencies not traditionally seen as part of the health provision for schools, have become established over recent years and will also contribute to the philosophy of extended services. The development of the school career service into the Connexions service has enabled different service providers to come together to support young people through their adolescent years. Personal advisors are based in schools and local communities to support young people in making choices about their future. This may be in relation to careers advice or it may provide a signposting service relating to those who have more complex needs and require more in-depth support to identify barriers to their learning, such as mental health problems, difficult family circumstances, drug abuse, homelessness or pregnancy.

Conclusion

Within the last 100 or so years there has been a vast array of legislation, policies, reports and guidance that have driven change in the way health is promoted and services provided for children and young people. Schools are seen as being one of the most natural places to promote health and the development of extended schools will also contribute to this. The importance of all agencies working with the school age population, collaborating in order to achieve the best outcomes for this client group has gained momentum over recent years. Bringing together health, education and social care could potentially provide a truly inclusive service promoting and protecting the health of all children and young people. There is also clear recognition that young people also gather in other places where health can be promoted. There are also those who do not attend school for a variety of reasons or who view school buildings as being authoritative places. Consequently, the health needs of these vulnerable young people are often neglected (DH, 2004b). Help must be delivered in partnership with other agencies, parents/carers and the young people themselves in order to provide a wide range of flexible services to meet their ever-increasing complex health needs and to reduce health inequalities. Many of the issues identified in this chapter are explored in more depth in other sections within this book.

References

Alcohol Concern (2007) *Alcohol Concern Quarterly Information and Research Bulletin*, available at http://www.alcoholconcern.org.uk/; accessed 6 August 2007.

Ball, J. and Pike, G. (2005) *School Nurses: Results from a Census Survey of RCN School Nurses in 2005*. Employment Research Ltd/RCN, London.

British Paediatric Association (BPA) (1995) *The Health Needs of School Age Children*. BPA, London.

Chamberlain, T., Lewis, K., Teeman, D. and Kendall, L. (2006) *What Is Happening in Extended Schools? Annual Survey of Trends in Education*. NFER for the Local Government Association. http://www.nfer.ac.uk/publications/other-publications/downloadable-reports/what-is-happening-on-extended-schools.cfm.

Court Committee Report (1976) *Fit for the Future: Report of the Committee on the Future of Child Health Services. Cmnd 6684*. HMSO, London.

Davies, P. (2007) *The NHS in the UK 2007/2008: A Pocket Book*. The NHS Confederation, London.

DeBell, D. and Jackson, P. (2000) *School Nursing Within the Public Health Agenda: a Strategy for Practice*. QNI, London.

Debell, D. and Tomkins, A. (2006) *Discovering the Future of School Nursing: the Evidence Base*. CPHVA, London.

Department for Children, Schools and Families (DCSF) (2007a) *Parents Know How*. Available at http://www.dcsf.gov.uk/; accessed 24 July 2007.

Department for Children, Schools and Families (DCSF) (2007b) *Extended Schools: Building on Experience*. DCSF Publications, Nottingham.

Department for Children, Schools and Families (2008) Raising Standards of School Meals. http://www.standards.dfes.gov.uk/forums/showflat.php?Cat=&Number=2048&page=0&view=collapsed&sb=5&o=&fpart=1; accessed 8 January 2008.

Department for Education and Skills (DfES) (2004a) *Healthy Living Blueprint for Schools*. DfES, London.

Department for Education and Skills (DfES). (2004b) *Extended Schools and Health Services – Working Together for Better Outcomes for Children and Families*. DfES publications, Nottingham.

Department for Education and Skills (DfES) (2005a) *Youth Matters: Next Steps – Something to Do, Somewhere to Go, Someone to Talk To*. DfES Publications, Nottingham.

Department for Education and Skills (DfES) (2005b) *National Healthy Schools Status: a Guide for Schools*. Stationery Office, London.

Department for Education and Skills (DfES) (2005c) *Higher Standards, Better Schools for All: More Choice for Parents and Pupils*. Stationery Office, London.

Department for Education and Skills(DfES) (2005d) *Extended Schools: Access to Opportunities and Services for All. A Prospectus*. DfES Publications, Nottingham.

Department for Education and Skills (DfES) (2005e) *Food in Schools*. Available at http://www.foodinschools.org.uk/; accessed 5 June 2007.

Department for Education and Skills (DfES) (2006a) *Planning and Funding Extended Schools: A Guide for Schools, Local Authorities and Their Partner Organisations*. DfES Publications, Nottingham.

Department for Education and Skills (DfES) (2006b) *What Do Extended Schools Mean for Health Professionals?* DfES Publications, Nottingham.

Department for Education and Skills (DfES) (2006c) *The Governance and Management of Extended Schools and Sure Start Children's Centres*. DfES Publications, Nottingham.

Department of Health/Department for Education and Skills (2003) *Every Child Matters*. DfES Publications, London.

Department of Health/Department for Education and Skills (2004) *Every Child Matters: Change for Children*. Stationery Office, London.

Department of Health (1989) *The Children Act*. HMSO, London.

Department of Health (1992) *The Health of the Nation*. HMSO, London.

Department of Health (1999a) *Healthy Schools Programme*. Stationery Office, London.

Department of Health (1999b) *Saving Lives: Our Healthier Nation*. Stationery Office, London.

Department of Health (2004a) *Choosing Health: Making Healthier Choices Easier*. Stationery Office, London.

Department Of Health (2004b) *The Children Act*. Stationery Office, London.

Department Of Health (2004c) *National Service Framework for Children, Young People and Maternity Services.* Stationery Office, London.

Department of Health (2004d) *Chief Nursing Officer's Review of the Nursing, Midwifery and Health Visiting Contribution to Vulnerable Children and Young People.* DH, London.

Department of Health (2006) *Looking for a School Nurse.* DH, London.

Education Act (2002) http://www.publications.parliament.uk/; accessed 16 November 2007.

Hall, D. and Elliman, D. (eds) (2003) *Health for All Children*, 4th edn. Oxford University Press, Oxford.

Harris, B. (1995) *The Health of the School Child: A History of the School Medical Service in England and Wales.* Open University Press, Buckingham,

Health Development Agency (2004) *Teenage Pregnancy: an Overview of Research Evidence.* HDA, York.

Health Protection Agency (2005) *Epidemiological Statistics Relating to Sexual Transmitted Infections.* Available at http://www.hpa.org.uk/infections/; accessed 8 August 2007.

Interdepartmental Committee on Physical Deterioration (1904) *Report of the Interdepartmental Committee on Physical Deterioration. Cmnd 2175. Vol. 1.* HMSO, London.

Johnson, S. (1977) For and against the Court Report. *Education*, pp. 248–9.

Laming, Lord (2003) *The Victoria Climbié Inquiry: Report of an Inquiry by Lord Laming.* Stationery Office, London.

Leff, S. and Leff, V. (1959) *The School Health Service.* Lewis, London.

Madge, N. and Franklin, A. (2003) *Change, Challenge and School Nursing.* National Children's Bureau, London.

McNalty, A. (1939) *Suggestions on Health Education: Board of Education for England.* HMSO, London.

Mental Health Foundation (2007) *Mental Health Information.* Available at http://www.mentalhealthfoundation.org/information/selfharm/; accessed 6 August 2007.

Naidoo, J. and Wills, J. (2000) *Health Promotion: Foundations for Practice*, 2nd edn. Baillière Tindall, London.

National Governors' Association (NGA) (2006) *Extended Schools – a Guide for Governors 1.* National Remodelling Team, Birmingham.

NHS Health and Social Care Information Centre (2006) *Public Health Statistics.* Available from http://www.ic.nhs.uk/; accessed 30 July 2007.

Nursing and Midwifery Council (2004) *Standards of Proficiency for Specialist Community Public Health Nurses.* Nursing and Midwifery Council, London.

Office for Standards in Education (Ofsted) (2005) *Personal, Social and Health Education in Secondary Schools.* HMI, London.

Office for Standards in Education (Ofsted) (2006) *Extended Services in Schools and Children's Centres*, Report 2609. http://www.dfes.gov.uk/assets/Internet_Content/Publications_Team/File_attachments/extended2609.pdf.

Spencer, N. (1998) *Progress in Community Health*, Vol. 2. Churchill Livingstone, Edinburgh.

Strehlow, M. S. (1987) *Nursing in Educational Settings.* Lippincott, London.

While, A. F. and Barriball, K. C. (1993) School Nursing: History, Present Practices and Possibilities Reviewed. *Journal of Advanced Nursing*, **18**, 1202–11.

Wilkin, A., White, R. and Kinder, K. (2003) *Towards Extended Schools: a Literature Review*. National Foundation for Educational Research, London.

Useful websites

The Healthy Schools Initiative: http://www.healthyschools.org.uk/

Every Child Matters: http://www.everychildmatters.gov.uk

Children Act 2004: http://www.opsi.gov.uk/acts

Department of Health: http:// ww.dh.gov.uk

Health Protection Agency: http://www.hpa.org.uk

Department for Children, Schools and Families: http://www.dcsf.gov.uk

CHAPTER 3

Assessing population health needs of children and young people

Joanne D. Bartley

Key themes

- Health is a complex concept and values attached to it from a children and young people perspective need to be understood.
- Needs are subjective and difficult to identify. The imposition of 'adult' perceptions can mislead priority identification with children.
- Assessment is a complex process which requires particular consideration with children and young people. Involvement is required at all stages, including priority setting.
- It is a challenge to fully engage children and young people in the process of developing a child-led service which reduces inequalities.

Introduction

The concept of delivering a needs-led NHS has been around for over a decade. The process of needs assessment, however, did not always involve asking communities directly about their needs but rather focused on secondary data collection and interpretation (Hawtin *et al.*, 1998). This is especially true where children and young people are concerned with the value of involving them in decisions about the delivery of services to meet their needs being an even newer concept. In general in the UK, the views of children and young people have not been valued, with the UK slow to adopt the full philosophy of the 1989 United Nations Convention on the Rights of the Child (UNICEF, 1990) which states:

> Children have the right to say what they think should happen, when adults are making decisions that affect them, and to have their opinions taken into account. (*Article 12, UNICEF, 1990*)

This was witnessed with the relatively late appointment of a children's commissioner in England in March 2005, several years behind its European counterparts. However, with the launch of the Children Act (Department of Health, [DH], 2004a), the *National Service Framework for Children, Young People and Maternity Services* (DH/Department for Education and Skills [DfES], 2004a) and subsequent strategies such as *Every Child Matters: Change for Children* (DH/DfES, 2004b) outlining plans for the reform of children's services, there is now a recognised need to engage children and young people in the commissioning of health and social services (Partridge, 2005). The Children's Commissioner for England is required by law to demonstrate that he is working in partnership with children and young people to assess their needs and plan appropriate services (DH, 2004a). In fact, all national strategies concerning children and young people are now focused on one common goal: to harmonise children's services to meet their needs and enable them to achieve their maximum potential (DH/DfES, 2006).

In order to achieve this goal, practitioners need to become skilled at assessing the needs of children and young people in the population before they can commission and deliver services which will support young people appropriately and effectively. This chapter therefore aims to explore the potentially complex process of 'health needs assessment' in relation to children and young people, an understanding of which should enable practitioners to develop those skills required.

> Health needs assessment is a systematic method for reviewing the health issues facing a population, leading to agreed priorities and resource allocation that will improve health and reduce inequalities. (NICE, 2005, p. 1)

This suggests that health needs assessment may not include public participation, as health data can be collected from secondary sources such as census information and public health research. However, the process does provide an opportunity for public involvement and this is identified as crucial to best practice. In particular, the consultation of children and young people in regard to their needs is central to health service reform in England (DH, 1998; DH/DfES, 2004b). The benefits of health needs assessment are then multiplied. As well as resulting in the more efficacious and appropriate allocation of resources, the process itself should support the development of team and partnership working across groups, including the community, and of knowledge, participation skills and confidence of the individuals and communities taking part.

This chapter is divided into three distinct sections, structured around the integral concepts of, 'health', 'needs' and 'assessment' and their relevance to children and young people. A variety of approaches to the concept of health in relation to children and young people is explored, and consideration is given to how these different models might be contrasted with how children and young people view health themselves, in particular the tendency for children and young people to focus on immediacy rather than considering the long-term health impact (Brewer, 2001). Concepts of empowerment and motivation are also discussed. Issues of power and control will also be explored in relation to parental involvement and influences. Frameworks for understanding health needs and methods for assessing those of children and young people are examined. The chapter concludes with a discussion of the challenges facing practitioners in health needs assessment, including tackling inequalities, accessing hard to reach groups and changing young people's views of health professionals and services in order to improve engagement (DH/DfES, 2004a).

Health as children and young people see it

Health is a concept which has had many definitions over the previous decades. The World Health Organization definition of 1946 is still often quoted as; 'not merely the absence of disease but complete physical, mental and social well-being'. This has been criticised for being an 'ideal' and therefore virtually impossible to achieve as well as omitting to consider other dimensions of relevance to people's well-being. Later attempts to conceptualise health have therefore taken a more holistic approach, encompassing a range of concepts including spirituality, emotional wellness and ultimately empowerment (WHO, 1986) and have also suggested that health is something to be enjoyed as a part of everyday life rather than a seemingly unattainable goal to be strived for (Seedhouse, 1986; Naidoo and Wills, 1994). This has resulted in a shift in philosophy in promoting health as witnessed in comparing the very different approaches taken in, for example, *The Health of the Nation* (DH, 1992) and *Choosing Health* (DH, 2004b). The former focused mainly on a biomedical model of individual pathology and behaviour as the cause of disease and hence the interventions proposed also focused on individuals. Over a decade later, *Choosing Health* encompassed a broader characterisation of health and its antecedents, including, for example, environmental and social factors (DH, 2004b). It also recognised the need to empower groups and individuals in order for them to make informed choices regarding their health, a concept intrinsic to the World Health Organization philosophy two decades ago (WHO, 1986). It is therefore best practice to invite people's views of their health needs and

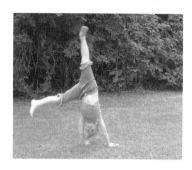 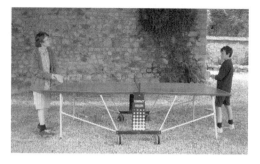

Physical exercise promotes health.

the types of services they believe will best meet them, as this process itself promotes the development of skills and confidence, which in turn, enables people
to make healthy choices and affect the environment around them (WHO, 1986;
Tones and Tilford, 1994).

Since the concept of 'health' itself remains a contentious one, it is crucial
when undertaking a health needs assessment that some agreement is sought
from those involved as to how health is perceived. The concept of 'health' will
necessarily inform the concept of 'health needs' and therefore a shared definition is vital to the process of measuring health in others in order to ensure
a clear focus for the assessment project. Therefore, in order to be truly successful at assessing the health needs of children and young people we must
understand what health means to them, otherwise the 'assessment tool', be it
a written questionnaire or set of focus group questions, will fail to generate a
valid picture of the group's health needs.

Generally, the cultural norm of 'health' has been defined by those in power
in society with scant attention paid to how populations and the individuals
within them interpret or define their own health needs (Naidoo and Wills,
2005). This is particularly true when considering children and young people
(Wright *et al.*, 2006). However, most recently, *Every Child Matters* (DH/DfES,
2004), defined five outcomes to be the right of all children, which were outlined in the Introduction.

These outcomes and the strategy itself were developed after consultation
with a range of contributors, including parents and children and young people.
The five outcomes are therefore indicative of children's and young people's
priorities although how much these were ameliorated by 'adult' views during
the process is uncertain. The Children's Commissioner for England was instru-
mental in setting up a two-day consultation event with 115 children who represented the views of their peers from around England. A range of methods, such
as art and drama, were used to elicit views. They identified the top priority for
children and young people as 'violence, abuse and bullying', with 'respect for
our views' as the second priority (11 million, 2007). The information from this

consultation exercise has been used to develop the '11 million 5 year plan': the commissioner's commitment to improving outcomes for all 11 million children and young people in England. This indicates that consultation with children and young people is possible and effective and can be used to inform policy development (Wright *et al.*, 2006).

Regardless of how children and young people define health, research suggests that whilst adults are mostly able to relate their current behaviour to future health outcomes this is not so with children and young people, whose psychology and stage of development tend to result in a focus on the very present (Brewer, 2001). Young adolescents in particular are prone to 'risk-taking behaviour', which often results in behaviours which are known to the individual to be 'unhealthy' but are nevertheless engaged in as a need to push the previously parentally controlled boundaries and to test the limits of their own power and control – alongside the basic human trait of curiosity! It is therefore imperative that children's and young people's attitudes to health are listened to and understood if health promoting interventions are to stand any chance of success with this specialised population group (DH, 2002). Partridge (2005) suggests that this requires a huge shift in many practitioners' attitudes towards power sharing with children and young people, as to truly engage young people practitioners need to 'surrender control' and allow children and young people 'to grow' in their ability to formulate and express their ideas effectively.

Needs

Once the concept of 'health' has been clarified, the next step in the health needs assessment process is to determine how 'needs' will be classified in order to provide a framework for analysis (Carey, 1999; Cavanagh and Chadwick, 2005).

There are many approaches to classifying needs, one of the most well known being Maslow's hierarchy of need (Maslow, 1987), which suggested that needs are 'incremental' and that as humans we need to satisfy basic needs, such as 'hunger, thirst and safety' before we progress to fulfil higher needs such as cognitive needs and the need for order and beauty. This would seem useful as a framework for younger children, who are driven by their need for food, drink and feeling safe and loved (Brewer, 2001). However, it may be a less useful tool for assessing adolescents' needs because, as was explored briefly earlier, adolescents are at a stage in their development where other motivators may be more relevant, for example, the need to 'fit in', or the need to take risks.

An alternative approach is Bradshaw's Taxonomy (Bradshaw, 1972). Although originally developed to classify sociological needs, the taxonomy has also been applied to classifying health needs. It suggests that needs fall into four categories: normative (defined by practitioners as the cultural 'norm'); comparative (a comparison with a similar group, again as defined by practitioners); felt needs (as 'felt' by individuals); and expressed needs, i.e. those which come to the attention of the practitioner. This is a useful tool when considering approaches to assessing the health needs of children and young people as it can be used to clarify the source of the need; e.g. are the needs identified the priorities of the practitioner – normative or comparative – or those of the clients – expressed? However, another issue of relevance here is whether the needs are those as expressed by the children and young people themselves or by their parents, carers and those who work with them, such as teachers, social workers or nurses. It is important that children and young people are not made to feel unduly responsible for decision making and the views of other significant adults and other relevant sources of information should in fact be 'triangulated' to ensure validity and reliability of assessment (DH, 2007). Assessment is discussed later.

A tension within all health needs assessment work, regardless of the target group, is the ethical consideration that needs to be given to a process which will potentially (and often) identify needs and raise expectations of interventions for which there is inadequate financial resource. Economists might argue that there are no 'absolute needs' – and health needs assessment simply 'raises unrealistic expectations' (Robinson and Elkan, 1996). This raises questions as to the purpose and focus of assessment and whether the focus of needs assessment should be where there is already evidence of effectiveness regarding a cost-effective intervention.

Assessment

The National Institute for Health and Clinical Excellence (NICE, 2005) identify five steps to health needs assessment, which are seen as:

- Getting started
- Identifying health priorities
- Assessing a health priority for action
- Action planning for change
- Moving on/project review
  (Cavanagh and Chadwick, 2005, p. 2)

Firstly it is important to clarify the aim of the health needs assessment: what it is hoped the assessment will achieve and for what purpose the information will be used. Health needs assessment is a time-consuming and complex process and there is little value in collecting data in an unfocused and haphazard manner. In order for the health needs assessment to be of use it needs a clear focus and structure. Part of this first step is to identify the information needed. This is where there needs to be clear definition of the population to be assessed, i.e. whether the entire practice population of children and young people is to be assessed or whether a subsection is chosen. A particular age group (e.g. 4 to 11 years) might be selected, or one school population, or indeed one age group within one school. The choice of population group will depend on the purpose of the health needs assessment and how the information gathered will be used. Once the population group has been defined, the detailed information required has to be decided. This is where a needs assessment framework can be useful.

The Common Assessment Framework (DfES, 2006) offers a model for assessment which focuses on three key influences: development of the child (young person); parents and carers; and family and environment. Although this was developed as a basis for assessment with individual children, it offers a comprehensive outline of the range of factors within each category (e.g. emotional warmth, family functioning and self-care skills) and could be used as the basis for developing a health needs assessment tool for use with population groups. More recently still, *Every Child Matters* (DH/DfES, 2004b) proposed the comprehensive outcomes framework based around the five key outcomes: be healthy; stay safe; enjoy and achieve; make a positive contribution; and achieve economic well-being. This includes consideration of a range of factors from basic physical, mental and sexual health, through enjoying school and recreational activities to taking part in decision making and enterprise opportunities. This would seem to provide an excellent framework for the exploration of children's and young people's needs in the current political and social climate, as the needs identified could be mapped to these categories, which are already seen as priorities nationally and locally. Once the framework for data collection has been decided, it is important to consider the philosophical approach that will be taken. Stevens and Gillam (1998) suggest that there are three separate but linked approaches.

- **Epidemiological** – based on the collecting of information about incidence, prevalence and the effectiveness of treatments.
- **Comparative** – which contrasts the services received in one area with those in another (as in Bradshaw's Taxonomy, 1972). It is based on uptake rates, service performance indicators and costs.
- **Corporate** – a structured collection of data on health care services and needs from a range of stakeholders, including healthcare professionals, patients and the wider public.

There are clearly costs and benefits to each approach. An epidemiological approach, whilst identifying disease trends, fails to elicit a consumer view of needs. Stevens and Gillam (1998) suggest that the comparative is also an incomplete assessment, as whilst providing information about relative need it fails to identify the precise need of either area. It is therefore suggested that a combination of all three approaches is taken in order to provide a comprehensive assessment from a wide range of data sources. This will provide both qualitative and quantitative data, each having its merits and providing differing perspectives. However, the approach taken will depend on the purpose of the health needs assessment.

In contrast to a guileless approach where a seemingly healthy population group is assessed with an open mind regarding their health needs, an alternative method is to identify a target group according to the presence of a pre-existing condition. For example, the needs of all children with asthma in an area or school might be assessed, or the needs of young carers. Hooper (1999) suggests a list of criteria that can be used to identify the focus of the enquiry. This includes the severity of the problem and the likelihood of a successful intervention. These criteria enable an approach which is mindful of the economists' argument against the 'open' exploration of need and focuses on the identification of needs that have proven cost-effective interventions (Billings and Cowley, 1995). Priorities identified in national and local strategies such as *Choosing Health* (DH, 2004b), the *National Service Framework for Children, Young People and Maternity Services* (DH/DfES, 2004a) and the local Children and Young People's Plan (DH/DfES, 2004a) can be used to direct an enquiry with a predetermined focus.

It can be seen from this discussion that it is crucial to begin the health needs assessment process with clearly defined aims and parameters if it is to result in a comprehensive and valid assessment of need (Cavanagh and Chadwick, 2005).

Data collection and analysis

A credible health needs assessment requires good quality data from reliable sources (Stevens and Gillam, 1998). Validity of the data can be enhanced by taking the 'combined' approach identified above: cross-checking data pertaining to the same issue from different sources. Wherever possible pre-collated data should be used, as this reduces the task. This might include data collected by others for research, Health Authority reports, and data compiled into profiles by other practitioners. However, it is crucial to ensure that the data collected is useful, not misleading, timely, accurate and complete. The methods used to involve children and young people in the data collection process needs to be evaluated to assess the validity of the views identified (Wright *et al.*, 2006).

However, for 'fresh' data, on a new group or related to a different need, a collection tool will need to be designed. Traditionally, schoolchildren's health needs have been assessed through a 'school profiling' exercise. Much of the data collected during this exercise was often taken from significant adults and school and medical records. Whilst this remains a useful and relevant method for data collection, it is suggested that this process should inform a small part of a much broader health needs assessment if the data gathered is to be a valid measure of children's and young people's views of their health needs. Many areas use Health Related Behaviour Questionnaires such as those devised by, and commissioned from, the Schools Health Education Unit, which are designed to elicit detailed information regarding all aspects of children's and young people's lifestyles. This information can then be used to inform service delivery. Some areas develop their own questionnaires, focusing their content on issues of concern locally (Coverdale and Lancaster, 2006). These can then be administered in the school setting with a captive audience and generally during school time with the agreement of the school. Discussion of how the information gathered will ultimately benefit the school is important, although confidentiality has to be carefully considered. An 'exam' environment is often used during data collection to increase the validity and confidentiality of the information. Questionnaires are generally anonymised and support needs to be obtained locally for the processing and feedback of the information. Any information given to the school should then be in anonymous form and provide an overview of trends rather than any information regarding individual pupil behaviours or concerns. One tension here may be that the mere process of completing the questionnaire may promote the needs for the young person to raise issues of concern with which they require support, and some mechanism for offering this has to be put in place. This might be a supplementary note to complete if a confidential one-to-one appointment is required, or simply identifying a time that a practitioner such as a school nurse, will be available for confidential one-to-one discussion.

However, this method, if used alone, potentially only records the health of children and young people attending school and therefore the needs of the wider school-age population will not be assessed. Ways of identifying and reaching marginalised groups, such as excluded pupils, disabled children and those children and young people in travelling families, need to be considered. This might include visiting youth groups, children's homes and youth detention centres. Partnership working with the agencies and practitioners involved with young people in a range of circumstances is therefore crucial (Danso *et al.*, 2003). Token participation of children and young people is insufficient and organisations need to establish a culture of continued engagement if they are to be effective (Danso *et al.*, 2003; DfES, 2004; Partridge, 2005; Wright *et al.*, 2006; 11 million, 2007). Traditional means of collecting data from clients may not be suitable for children and young people, and other techniques such as drama and art might be more appropriate. Very young children can be asked to draw a picture of the issue that worries them most; older children might express their views through the development of short dramatic pieces or game playing (11 million, 2007). Discussion groups and consultation events might be used to influence local service delivery, whereas websites can be utilised to seek children's and young people's views on broader policy decisions (Kirby *et al.*, 2003). Practitioners may need to develop more skills in these areas or develop new working partnerships with those who already have these skills (Partridge, 2006). Clearly practitioners also need to be skilled in their communication and partnership approaches with children and young people and their families (Bannister, 2001). Not all families are readily able to express their needs and a great deal of work may need to be done to empower them to develop the skills and confidence necessary before the process of assessment can begin.

The mechanism for data analysis should have been determined at the beginning of the process. Computer software packages may be available through local Trust and Public Health departments; some qualitative data may be processed manually (see Bowling, 1997 and Parahoo, 1997 for discussion of these methods).

Defining local need and addressing local priorities

A key part of health needs assessment and an essential skill for those working to address children's and young people's needs is priority setting. This should be seen as integral to the health needs assessment process, as the exercise has little value unless its results are utilised to develop services to meet need. However, agreeing priorities within competing agendas can be fraught with difficulty. The health needs assessment should map existing needs against a profile of local services; this highlights 'unmet' needs. As it is unlikely that funding exists to address all the needs, a framework for priority setting should be agreed with all partners, including children and young people, as it is crucial that some degree of consensus is reached regarding priorities (Steven and Gillam, 1998).

Practitioners require an understanding of the national NHS agenda, local 'Children and Young People's Plans' (DfES, 2005) and resource management in order for priorities to be set within this context. The priorities identified have to be matched against the current target areas for children's and young people's health, which are: childhood obesity; mental health; sexual health; accidents; and substance misuse (DH/DfES, 2004a; DH, 2004b; DH/DfES, 2006). Complex ethical issues and tensions exist within the present culture of performance and outcome measures and 'value for money' (Seedhouse, 1998; Mitton and Donaldson, 2004) and whilst practitioners and organisations are required to demonstrate that they are making an explicit contribution to meeting pre-identified targets and priorities for health improvement, children's and young people's priorities may be different. However, the Children's Commissioner for England is committed to listening to children and young people and ensuring that their views are represented across all government decision making. Over time, this will hopefully result in national policy which more accurately affects the views of young people, particularly in regard to their health. In the meantime, those working with children and young people have to carefully weigh their organisational priorities against those needs identified and hopefully reach a reasonable compromise.

Several approaches to priority setting exist, but a common element is the use of a 'grid' (Honigsbaum *et al.*, 1995; Coast *et al.*, 1996; Harris, 1997; Ewles and Simnett, 1999). Everyone involved in the health needs assessment process should agree a set of criteria, e.g. national and local priorities, level of need, severity of health impact, effectiveness of intervention and resource available. This leads to the making of a cross-referenced grid listing needs and scoring them for each criterion, in which the tensions are immediately evident. Prioritising the criteria and scoring the needs against each can be a difficult and subjective task. It is therefore important to agree the scoring system before the process of prioritising begins. Evidence demonstrating effectiveness can also be difficult to achieve (Mitton and Donaldson, 2004), particularly with children and young people, where interventions are often seeking to minimise health risks over the long term. Short-term goals also have to be set in order to satisfy commissioners of the worth of the input (Naidoo and Wills, 1994; Ewles and Simnett, 1999).

The final stages of the health needs assessment process are to draw up action plans and evaluate (Cavanagh and Chadwick, 2005). The action taken will depend on what is prioritised and may include revision of existing services, staff training, parental involvement or designing a new service. Planning and evaluation frameworks exist to aid this process and can be accessed through the following sources: Naidoo and Wills (1994), Ewles and Simnett (1999), Tones and Tilford (1994) and Cavanagh and Chadwick (2005).

The challenges

In conclusion it can be seen that the process of health needs assessment with children and young people is a challenging one (Partridge, 2005). Nonetheless it is essential to the philosophy of children's and young people's services and vital to achieving best practice (DfES, 2004; 11 million, 2007). Needs assessment is a key part of the government's inequalities agenda and it is therefore crucial that practitioners develop the knowledge and skills necessary to engage with all children and young people, especially vulnerable and marginalised groups, to facilitate the identification of needs and the provisions of appropriate services (Bannister, 2001; DH/DfES, 2004b, 2006). An understanding of children's and young people's perceptions of health and illness and their concerns regarding their futures is fundamental to the assessment process (DH, 2002). The next challenge lies in designing appropriate methods for data collection. Children and young people often enjoy expressing themselves creatively and modes such as artwork and drama are often very successful in motivating and engaging young people (11 million, 2007). However, the ability of children and young people to engage in more traditional methods of participation, such as questionnaires and focus groups, should not be underestimated, as their contribution often exceeds what is traditionally expected of them (Partridge, 2005). This supports the notion that a complete shift in organisational culture to one which routinely values and involves children and young people in all decision-making processes is required if successful participation is to result (Partridge, 2005; Wright *et al.*, 2006).

Health needs assessment and priority setting in the current climate is beset with tension and ethical conflict (Mitton and Donaldson, 2004; Stevens and Gillam, 1998). It is therefore imperative that children and young people are involved in all stages of the process, including priority setting, in order that these tensions can be considered and reduced (Wright *et al.*, 2006). Health needs assessment should then result in better use of resources to reduce inequalities in children's and young people's health (DfES, 2005).

References

Bannister, A. (2001) Entering the child's world: communicating with children to assess their needs. In: *The Child's World: Assessing Children in Need* (ed. J. Horwarth). Jessica Kingsley, London.

Billings, J. and Cowley, S. (1995) Approaches to community needs assessment: a literature review. *Journal of Advanced Nursing*, **22**, 721–30.

Bowling, A. (1997) *Research Methods in Health*. Open University press, Buckingham.

Bradshaw, J. (1972) The concept of social need. *New Society*, **30**, 640–3.

Brewer, S. (2001) *A Child's World*. Headline, London.

Carey, L. (1999) Using health profiling as a tool for needs assessment. *Nursing Times Learning Curve*, **2**(12), 6–7.

Cavanagh, S. and Chadwick, K. (2005) *Health Needs Assessment: A Practical Guide*. National Institute for Health and Clinical Excellence, London.

Coast, J., Donovan, J. and Frankel, S. (1996) *Priority Setting: The Healthcare Debate.* Wiley, Chichester.

Coverdale, G. and Lancaster, K. (2006) HNA – the theory gap recedes. *Journal of Community Nursing*, **20**(8), 10–16.

Danso, C., Greaves, H., Howell, S., Ryan, M., Sinclair, R. and Tunnard, J. (2003) *The Involvement of Children and Young People in Promoting Change and Enhancing the Quality of Social Care.* National Children's Bureau, London.

Department for Education and Skills (2005) *Children and Young People's Plan.* Stationery Office, London.

Department for Education and Skills (2006) *The Common Assessment Framework: Practitioners' Guide.* Stationery Office, London.

Department of Health/Department for Education and Skills (2004a) *The National Service Framework for Children, Young People and Maternity Services.* DfES, London.

Department of Health/Department for Education and Skills (2004b) *Every Child Matters: Change for Children.* DH, London.

Department of Health/Department for Education and Skills (2006) *School Nurse Practice Development Resource Pack.* DfES, London

Department of Health (1998) *Quality Protects.* Stationery Office, London.

Department of Health (1992) *The Health of the Nation.* HMSO, London.

Department of Health (2002) *Listening, Hearing and Responding.* DH, London.

Department of Health (2004a) *The Children Act.* Stationery Office, London.

Department of Health (2004b) *Choosing Health.* Stationery Office, London.

Department of Health (2007) *Improving the Quality and Outcomes for Services to Children and Young People Through Effective Commissioning: a Self-assessment Tool for Commissioners.* DH, London.

Ewles, L. and Simnett, I. (1999) *Promoting health*, 4th edn. Harcourt-Brace, London.

Harris, A (ed.) (1997) *Needs to Know: a Guide to Health Needs Assessment for Primary Care.* Churchill Livingstone, London.

Hawtin, M., Hughes, G. and Percy-Smith, J. (1998) Community *Profiling: Auditing Social Needs.* Open University Press, Buckingham.

Honigsbaum, F., Calltrop, J., Ham, C. and Holmstron, S. (1995) *Priority Setting Processes for Healthcare.* Radcliffe Medical Press, Oxford.

Hooper, J. (1999) Health needs assessment: helping change happen. *Community Practitioner*, **72**(9), 286–8.

Kirby, P., Lanyon, C., Cronin, K. and Sinclair, R. (2003) *Building a Culture of Participation.* DfES, London.

Maslow, A. (1987) *Motivation and Personality*, 3rd edn. Harper & Row, New York.

Mitton, C. and Donaldson, C. (2004) *Health Care Priority Setting: Principles, Practice and Challenges. Cost Effectiveness and Resource Allocation, 2,* http://resource-allocation.co./content/2/1/3; accessed 19 December 2007.

Naidoo, J. and Wills, J. (1994) *Health Promotion: Foundations for Practice.* Baillière Tindall, London.

Naidoo, J. and Wills, J. (2005) *Public Health and Health Promotion: Developing Practice*, 2nd edn. Baillière Tindall, London.

National Institute for Clinical Health Excellence (2005) *Health Needs Assessment.* http://www.nice.org.uk/aboutnice/whoweare/aboutthehda/hdapublications/ health_needs_assessment_a_practical_guide.jsp.

Parahoo, K. (1997) *Nursing Research: Principles, Process and Issues.* MacMillan, London.

Partridge, A. (2005) Children and young people's inclusion in public decision-making. *Support for Learning,* **20**(4).

Robinson, J. and Elkan, R. (1996) *Health Needs Assessment – Theory and Practice.* Churchill Livingstone, London.

Seedhouse, D. (1986) *Health: the Foundations for Achievement.* John Wiley, Chichester.

Stevens, A. and Gillam, S. (1998) Needs assessment: from theory to practice. *British Medical Journal,* **316**, 1448–52.

Tones, K. and Tilford, S. (1994) *Health Promotion: Effectiveness, Efficiency and Equity,* 2nd edn. Chapman & Hall, London.

UNICEF (1990) *1989 United Nations Convention on the Rights of the Child.* UNICEF.

World Health Organization (1986) *The Ottawa Charter for Health Promotion.* WHO, Geneva.

Wright, P., Turner, C., Clay, D. and Mills, H. (2006) *Practice Guide 6: Involving Children and Young People in Developing Social Care.* Social Care Institute for Excellence, London. http://www.scie.org.uk/publications/practiceguides/practiceguide06/index.asp; accessed on 19 December 2007.

11 million (2007) *The Five Year Plan: April 2007–March 2012. London.* Office of the Commissioner for Children in England. http://www.11million.org.uk/; accessed 21 December 2007.

Useful website

Schools Health Education Unit: http://www.sheu.org.uk/.

CHAPTER 4

Models of health promotion in action: what works?

Penny Farrelly

Key themes

- Health promotion models and theories
- The importance of developing health promotion strategies using theoretical frameworks
- Practical examples of health promotion initiatives that demonstrate different theories in action

Introduction

School and community nurses are among the professionals most concerned with children's well-being and traverse all the environments of the child, that is, the home, the school and the wider community as well as connecting with the multi-sectoral nature of the service provision for young people. They are also the nursing professionals with responsibility for addressing the needs of children through childhood, providing an opportunity to develop an in-depth knowledge of individual and family needs over time. Additionally, they have the expertise to provide comprehensive responses to complex health needs as they combine clinical knowledge relating to the school-age population with an understanding of the connection between the social determinants of health and delivery of effective health promotion, and it is this aspect that we are concerned with here. This chapter will explore the use of theory in support of health promotion. There are a number of different perspectives used by health promoters which influence the ways in which they approach their work. Readers will be encouraged to think about ways in which a range of theoretical approaches to health promotion can be applied to and integrated within their role.

Using theory to organise practice

Most health promotion theories are derived from the behaviour and social sciences. They borrow from disciplines such as psychology and sociology and from activities such as a consumer behaviour and marketing. Therefore it is easy to understand that health promotion is concerned not just with the behaviour of individuals, but with the ways in which society is organised and the policies and organisational structures that underpin society. Many of the theories used in health promotion have not been highly developed, nor rigorously tested and for these reasons they should be more accurately described as models (Bunton and MacDonald, 2002).

Clearly, one does not approach a client or issue and start thinking about which theoretical framework one wants to apply to a particular situation; this would reinforce the theory–practice dichotomy, and seems abstract and false. It is useful, however, to work out whether theorists have made any useful contribution that can support or inform aspects of practice before setting out to target a specific topic.

The simplest way of thinking about models is to see them as a way in which theorists reduce their thinking to the bare bones of their ideas so that they present a diagrammatic portrait or picture of the priorities and issues they envisage in carrying out health promotion. The same can be said of nursing models, which are often used as a checklist to ensure that nothing is missed out when planning patient care. Health promotion models are best used when the health promotion initiative has been properly planned so that it follows the full cycle of development; that is: planning, intervention, reflection and evaluation. They do not readily lend themselves to the kind of health promotion that many health care professionals find themselves engaging in where they deal with a situation that arises 'off the cuff' without having the advantage of planning for it.

Some models lend themselves to working with individuals and Ewles and Simnett (2003) and Downie *et al.* (1996) in particular spring to mind here. Others, such as Beattie (1991) and Tones and Tilford (2001), take more of a public health approach and attempt to devise a strategy to deal with the underlying structures that affect health. Table 4.1 offers a useful outline of the relationship between key health promotion approaches.

One can see that both school and community nursing fit well between health education and individual empowerment. One could argue that governments (particularly the pre-1997 Conservative one) might be particularly interested in behaviour change and in encouraging individuals to take responsibility for their own health, so this approach is focused much more on individuals and involves the use of particular approaches:

Table 4.1 Four levels of health promotion.

1. Health education: giving information

Individual/community/national/international

Individual information is given in schools and health clinics to children, young people and parents.

Community or public meetings can give information to groups, for example on safety of immunisations; practitioners can run groups such as parenting.

Health information freely available via information technology; individuals better informed about their health than ever before.

Giving information gives people *knowledge* to make informed decisions.

2. Individual empowerment: enabling choice

Knowledge is not necessarily enough to make healthy choices.

Children and young people, and their parents may not be able to make those choices due to their family circumstances.

Individual empowerment intends to build self-esteem, self-efficacy and improve self awareness. Self esteem programmes are becoming more common in schools as well as parenting courses.

Individuals empowerment concepts build the SKILLS needed for making healthy choices.

3. Community development: group action

Personal knowledge and skills are important, but group action may initiate change more effectively.

Working in partnership across sectors will bring pressure on organisations to change. For example, setting up a health drop in will require local action with schools, pupils parents, governors, health and social sectors.

Community groups can also lobby parliament for more national change if motivated to act. Can be negative, for example parents protesting about the triple MMR vaccine in the late '90s.

Group activity provides *action*.

4. Political action: structural adjustment

Top-down approaches to health promotion through government legislation are led by many influences.

Healthy public policy benefits society because health is seen as a major determinant of socio-economic stability.

National scandals and tragedies such as the death of Victoria Climbié stimulate huge change to policy. Structural adjustment in terms of children and children's services have led to new government departments and a children's health agenda (*Every Child Matters*).

The smoking ban is good example of political action which aims to give individuals no choice.

Political action provides *power*.

- Medical
- Behaviour change
- Educational
- Client-centred or empowerment
- Social change or radical

Choosing a theoretical framework

Over the past two decades theorists have refined and reviewed their work so that where they once focused directly on modification of individual behaviour many now recognise the importance of influencing and changing a broad range of social, economic and environmental factors that influence health alongside individual behavioural choices. This can be seen in post-1997 Labour-led policy.

Taking this approach, and as pointed out by Davies and MacDowall (2006), health promotion operates at several different levels:

- Individual
- Community
- Organisation
- Nation

The level of the intervention may help one to choose the approach. Taking the example of a programme aimed at improving the uptake of a school counselling service one can see that interventions could be implemented at the level of the individual, the community, the organisation of services and at the national level. This might involve:

- Education to inform and motivate individual children about the service
- Facilitation of community debate to change perceptions concerning child and adolescent mental health
- More widely available services
- Financial incentives for doctors to increase their contact with young people

Given the level of an intervention (individual, group, organisation or nation), no one theorist can provide all the solutions to the health needs. It follows therefore that the models are not written in tablets of stone and should be adapted to suit particular needs. In order to be useful, theories must be easy to understand and adaptable to many different situations. All of them should enable effective planning of interventions at the appropriate level in order to address a health need or issue.

This chapter will look at the following concepts:

■ Individual – the Health Belief Model (Nutbeam and Harris, 2004)
■ Community – Beattie (1991)
■ Nation – Social marketing (NSMC, 2005)

These models will be discussed and their practical application explored using specific examples from practice.

Individual focus – the Health Belief Model

The Health Belief Model (HBM) is a psychological model that attempts to explain and predict health behaviours. This is done by focusing on the attitudes and beliefs of individuals. The HBM was first developed in the 1950s by social psychologists working in the US Public Health Services. The model was developed in response to the failure of a free tuberculosis (TB) health screening program. Since then, the HBM has been adapted to explore a variety of long- and short-term health behaviours, including risky sexual behaviour and the transmission of HIV/AIDS.

The HBM is designed to explain health behaviour by explaining the thought processes that one goes through when making decisions about health and health care. Fundamentally, the model suggests that the likelihood of an individual taking action for a health problem is based on the interaction between four types of belief. The model predicts that individuals will take action to protect or promote health if:

■ they see themselves to be susceptible to a condition or problem
■ they believe it will have potentially serious consequences
■ they believe a course of action is available which will reduce their susceptibility or minimise the consequences
■ they believe that the benefits of taking action will outweigh the costs or barriers.

The model can be illustrated diagrammatically as in Table 4.2.

An example of this model in use would be the initiatives applied during the winter of 2004 that Primary Care Trusts (PCTs) across London carried out to protect thousands of primary school-age children against measles, mumps and rubella. At that time, in London, the uptake of vaccinations among children at five years of age for the first dose of the MMR vaccine was 80%, and coverage of the second dose only 58%. A second dose ensures a child is fully protected from these childhood diseases (DH, 2006). The World Health Organization

Table 4.2 The MMR example: applying the Health Belief Model. (Adapted from Nutbeam and Harris, 2004)

Perceived susceptibility

Parents need information about how susceptible their children are to contracting measles in the first place. What is the risk if they do not have the vaccine? They need this information from reliable sources with accurate information.

Perceived seriousness

If the child does contract measles, what is the consequence of this weighed against the perceived problems with the MMR triple vaccine?

Perceived benefits

What is the benefit to having the MMR vaccine?

Parents are not always interested in the concept of herd immunity, they are more concerned with their own child's health.

Perceived barriers

Access to health services and accurate information may be a barrier such as language difficulties, families living in isolated areas, asylum seekers etc.

Perceived threat

Research which introduces doubt to the efficacy of the MMR vaccine provides a powerful threat to action.

Outcome expectations

The outcome of having the vaccine will need to be balanced by parents against the outcome of not having it. The choice that parents make on behalf of their children hinges on their outcome expectation.

Self-efficacy (perceived ability to carry out recommended action)

Parents may feel unable to make decisions given the conflicting advice. They may not be confident about their decision, particularly as it is for another individual, albeit their child. They may choose to avoid the decision.

recommends immunity levels of around 95% of the population to prevent outbreaks of disease (WHO, 2008).

It was felt that thousands of children in London were at risk of contracting measles, mumps and rubella following several years of decline in the numbers that were protected by the MMR vaccine. Because of the fall in the uptake of vaccinations, and the risk to public health, it was considered vital that the issue was addressed, particularly as uptake of other vaccinations may have been affected. Therefore, from November 2004, PCTs, working with the health protection units from the Health Protection Agency (HPA) in London, implemented a range of measures to improve uptake. These included especially arranged 'catch-up' sessions held both in schools and general practice settings (DH, 2004a).

Efforts to offer catch-up vaccinations to primary schoolchildren were considered particularly effective in reducing the risk of wider community outbreaks, as primary school-age children have many more social contacts than preschoolers, and often pass the infection to younger siblings. From that November, participating schools sent out information to parents and an invitation to have their child vaccinated at school if they had not yet received the recommended two doses of the MMR vaccine. Parents were provided with a consent form on which to indicate whether or not they wished to have their child vaccinated.

In terms of the application of the HBM, for the offer of the MMR vaccination to be taken up parents had to believe that their children might be susceptible to one of the three diseases covered by the vaccine. They had to believe that if they did contract one of the diseases that the child was likely to be severely ill as a result. Therefore, it was important that the advertising campaign stressed the fact that measles can lead to encephalitis and death in one in a thousand infected children and that mumps can cause sensori-neural deafness and sub-fertility (DH, 2006). This emphasises the complications of the diseases, which can be avoided by having the vaccine.

It was important that parents believed the vaccine to be effective in preventing the children from developing the diseases and that the vaccine itself posed no risk to health. We are aware, of course, that this is what had led to the poor uptake rate in the first place. The opinion of the public that the vaccine would *cause no harm* was crucial, but this view was challenged by research presented by Wakefield *et al.*, 1998). Wakefield suggested a link between children developing autism and bowel problems and the MMR vaccine.

This has since been challenged and no independent study has been able to replicate the results of the Wakefield study (BMA, 2008). The uptake for the MMR vaccine increased during 2006/2007 to 85% in the UK, and although still short of the 95% recommended by the World Health Organization (WHO, 2008), it is an improvement as public confidence grows in the triple vaccine (BMA, 2008).

One can see that the HBM works very well as a way of explaining behaviour in this type of situation – it is also used to explain the thought processes behind the decision to attend or not for screening procedures. The final area that the model covers is that of self-efficacy. People must feel able to make a decision themselves that they can then act upon with confidence, so the government has spent a lot of money ensuring that information has been freely available concerning the benefits of vaccination.

Community focus – Beattie's model

Beattie's model (1991) presents four quadrants of activity derived from two axes on a grid (Figure 4.1). The vertical axis represents modes of intervention that range from authoritarian, top down, expert-led interventions to bottom-up, negotiated, participatory approaches to health promotion. It could be suggested that nurses have traditionally been associated with fairly authoritarian, top-down approaches, but they also have the potential to play an important role in more participatory forms of health promotion, as we shall see. The horizontal axis represents the focus of activities ranging from interventions targeting individuals to those focused on tackling the social determinants of health. Again, the nurse's role is often seen to fit more comfortably with a focus on individuals despite a shifting emphasis to collective approaches within the

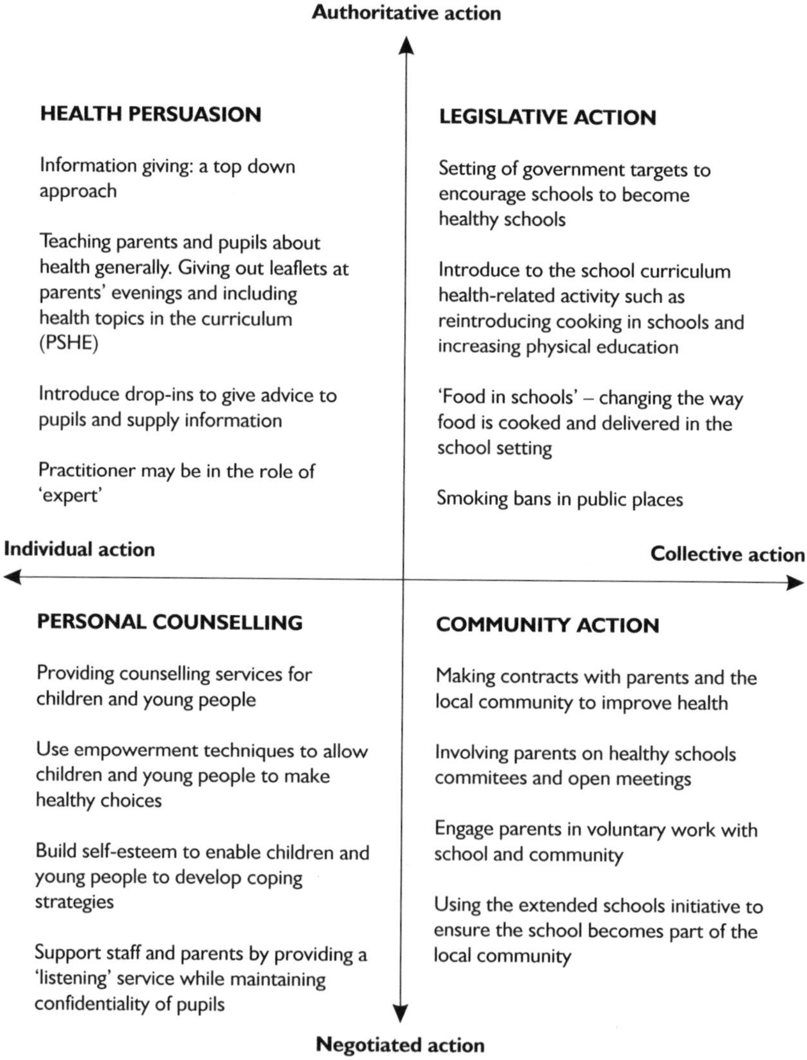

Authoritative action

HEALTH PERSUASION

Information giving: a top down approach

Teaching parents and pupils about health generally. Giving out leaflets at parents' evenings and including health topics in the curriculum (PSHE)

Introduce drop-ins to give advice to pupils and supply information

Practitioner may be in the role of 'expert'

LEGISLATIVE ACTION

Setting of government targets to encourage schools to become healthy schools

Introduce to the school curriculum health-related activity such as reintroducing cooking in schools and increasing physical education

'Food in schools' – changing the way food is cooked and delivered in the school setting

Smoking bans in public places

Individual action ←————————————————————→ **Collective action**

PERSONAL COUNSELLING

Providing counselling services for children and young people

Use empowerment techniques to allow children and young people to make healthy choices

Build self-esteem to enable children and young people to develop coping strategies

Support staff and parents by providing a 'listening' service while maintaining confidentiality of pupils

COMMUNITY ACTION

Making contracts with parents and the local community to improve health

Involving parents on healthy schools commitees and open meetings

Engage parents in voluntary work with school and community

Using the extended schools initiative to ensure the school becomes part of the local community

Negotiated action

Figure 4.1 The 'Healthy Schools Initiative': using Beattie's model of health promotion. (Adapted from: Naidoo and Wills, 2000)

field of health promotion. Within Beattie's model there are four spheres of health promotion activity:

- health persuasion
- legislative action
- personal counselling
- community development

Health persuasion

Health persuasion activities involve an expert-led top-down approach implying a rather paternalistic attitude and that the practitioner knows best. Its primary objective is to convince individuals to change their behaviour to adopt a healthier lifestyle. Epidemiological evidence is likely to be used to target high-risk patients and health issues. A health persuasion intervention is often based on the giving of information about behaviour (for instance trying to persuade a patient to undertake some healthier behaviour such as giving up smoking or taking more exercise) by outlining to them what the benefits to their health might be. Clearly it is likely to be popular with staff working in hospital settings where patients are admitted suffering from particular health problems and who may be amenable to changes in their behaviour. They may be considered a 'captive audience'.

This approach may be limited in its long-term effects and does not take into account the client's readiness or ability to change behaviour; it also does not explore the issues within the context of the client's life and circumstances or address the wider social and economic determinants of health.

Legislative action

Legislative action is also concerned with changing behaviour but through the benevolent actions of the state or an organisation. This approach includes actions to bring about changes to national legislation, the development of national, local or organisational policies and supportive environments for health and the provision of adequate resources for health to support national programmes. Such actions aim to make healthier choices easier. While interventions at this level can encourage change, universal measures are often unable to meet the specific needs of all minority groups or individuals within a population (for example the smoking ban in public places).

Community development

Community development is committed to bottom-up, community-led participatory approaches and seeks to bring about change at local, regional and national levels. Such interventions are based on the empowerment of communities to identify and prioritise their own needs, to work together to seek solutions to those needs and to implement change as part of an ongoing process. The community involved may be a geographical community, but may also be a community defined by culture, interest or identity.

Advocates of community development (Ledwith, 2005) argue that interventions are therefore more relevant, create a sense of ownership and are more likely to be effective and sustainable. It always has certain key aims which are:

- To combat social exclusion
- To promote participation and
- To encourage people to acquire new skills

The community development process is based on principles of social justice and equity, and requires professionals to be led by the communities they work with. This becomes a potentially radical approach to health promotion which may present certain challenges for some, particularly if the priorities of the community do not match those of the professional or current health policy agendas. Community development can be a complex process that requires time and trust in order to develop relationships, networks and effective ways of working. Goals may be initially unclear, become clarified and change with time. It is also often an inter-sectoral approach that involves partnerships with other statutory and voluntary bodies. Effective community development begins with a process of empowerment through critical consciousness-raising where individuals and communities are encouraged to begin questioning and challenging the social justice of their situation. Nurses have the potential to be involved in this process with both individuals and communities by raising awareness of the wider factors that determine health choices. This can then contribute to a collective action at a wider community level.

Personal counselling

Interventions within this theme are also led by, or negotiated with, the client and are based on one-to-one work. The role of the nurse in this situation is to listen to the client and work to empower that individual to make the changes they feel they need to make. This might involve problem-solving strategies and skills development tools, as well as confidence and self-esteem building. Such approaches can be used either to promote positive health and well-being or to prevent ill health through disease management. Developing partnerships with patients and their family in the management of long-term conditions may be an example of such a technique. One of the key aspects of this approach is the importance of ensuring that the patient and family are able to carry on independently once that support has been withdrawn (see Chapter 10).

Beattie's model is useful for helping to select a mix of approaches that will make up a programme of health promotion or project. The model gives an indication that health is embedded in the context of the socio-cultural and political framework; there is a tension between different value positions about power, knowledge responsibility and autonomy. It is not therefore simply a question of choosing the strategy but also considering all of these other factors that may limit and influence the aims of the intervention.

The strength of Beattie's model lies in the fact that it recognises that one approach chosen from one of the four quadrants will not be enough to bring about a positive change in health for clients. The need for a particular intervention will change with time and may involve other factors along the way. The healthy schools campaign (DfES, 1999) is a good example that demonstrates all of the elements of Beattie's model. As the homepage for 'Healthy Schools' says:

> Healthy Schools help children and young people to reach their potential
> by building on a solid foundation of health to do better in learning and
> in life.

The programme takes an holistic approach to health and well-being, involving not just the pupils but the whole school community, from parents to governors to school staff, in improving their health and their happiness and getting the most out of life. The legislative action quadrant of the model is evident as the Government has set a target that all schools will be participating in the National Healthy Schools Programme by 2009 and that 75% of schools will have achieved National Healthy School Status (Nutbeam, 2003) (see Chapter 5).

The community development quadrant is addressed by the way in which is the whole school approach is central to the National Healthy Schools Programme. Achieving National Healthy School Status recognises that being healthy is not just about children and young people, but is about the whole school community. It is not just what happens in the curriculum, it is about the entire school day, through to after-school activities. Through adopting this approach it is hoped to achieve full engagement with the school community and to secure sustainable improvements.

The health persuasion and personal counselling components of the model can be seen in some of the elements of the whole school approach, particularly in those of:

- Teaching and learning
- Giving children and young people a voice
- Provision of pupil support services
- Staff professional development needs, health and welfare
- Partnerships with parents/carers and local communities

National focus – the social marketing model

Not a theory in itself, social marketing draws on other theories such as the transtheoretical model (Prochaska and DiClemente, 1992) and the social cognitive theory (Bandura, 2000), both widely used as a basis for understanding individual behaviour, as well as the Health Belief Model already explored and exchange theory (Houston and Gassenheimer, 1987), which suggests that we are all striving to improve our lot. In order to increase consumers' readiness to change, social marketers must provide them with something beneficial in exchange. In terms of children and young people, this will involve developing understanding of the young person in society and the influences on the choices they make as they grow up.

There has been a growing recognition over recent years that we need to concentrate on focusing our efforts in health promotion on those that make policies and pass legislation to improve health, thus 'moving upstream'. Social marketing came to prominence in England with the publication of the public health White Paper *Choosing Health* (DH, 2004b). Under the heading 'Marketing Health', the Government described how they took evidence from, 'people who help make the less healthy choices the sexy ones – marketers and advertisers' (p. 21). These professionals told the Government that:

> the power of 'social marketing', marketing tools applied to social good, could be used to build public awareness and change behaviour, making behaviour that harms health less attractive and encouraging behaviour that builds health

The Government has since established a National Social Marketing Centre for Excellence (NSMC) to increase understanding and use of social marketing at national, regional and local level. The Department of Health has defined social marketing as:

> the systematic application of marketing concepts and techniques to achieve specific behavioural goals relevant to a social good.

In health-related social marketing the social good is defined as:

> improving health and reducing health inequalities (NSMC, 2005, p. 31)

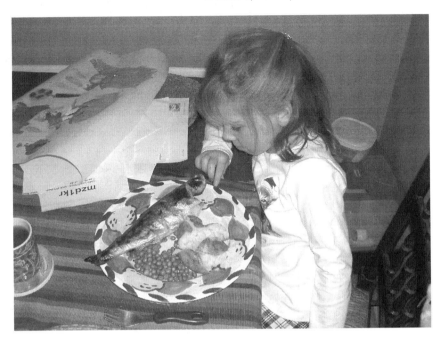

Health promotion covers a variety of issues including nutrition.

The Wanless Review (2004) focused on the public health and inequalities challenge across Government. Improving health and reducing health inequalities is acknowledged as a major challenge that will only be achieved if we are able to encourage a step change in what we do, harnessing the potential of all sectors. Simply doing more of what we have been doing, even if we do this better, is unlikely to achieve the goals. Social marketing is considered by the Government to be the answer to changing our approach and achieving much better health for the nation.

Social marketing can be considered as a set of concepts and principles to inform and enhance the development of effective policy, strategy and implementation; that is, as a frame of reference or a mindset to help examine, understand and provide insight into issues and also enhance impact and effectiveness. It is also a specific intervention method or planned process to support implementation by providing a systematic process to achieve targeted behavioural goals as a specific social marketing intervention.

Growing evidence and experience, particularly from countries like Canada, Australia and the US, show that when social marketing is applied effectively, and in the appropriate context, it can be a powerful tool for achieving tangible and measurable impact on behaviours (Hastings and Haywood, 2002). Improving the level of understanding and application of social marketing is critical if we are to achieve real and measurable impacts on young people's health across a range of different policy and practice agendas.

Ultimately, health promotion is concerned with influencing behaviour. Therefore, it seems sensible to take a lesson from the commercial world of advertising and media and use similar strategies to achieve this aim. Clearly we can criticise this activity when it does harm, as in the case of the tobacco industry, but we should be prepared to learn from it when the opportunity exists to do good. There are six key features and concepts crucial to understanding social marketing:

1. **Customer or consumer orientation**

   A strong 'customer' orientation with importance attached to understanding where customers are starting form, their knowledge, attitudes and beliefs, along with the social context in which they live. In this case, the customer is the young person with a particular set of developmental needs, 'rites of passage' and external influences such as family, school and peers. Where the young person is perhaps at an early stage of knowledge acquisition and open to new 'marketing' strategies and ideas, selling health as an option rather than unhealthy activity may be the way forward, and those working in health and education are in a good position to achieve this.

2. **Behaviour and behavioural goals**

   Clear focus on understanding existing behaviour and key influences on it, alongside developing clear behavioural goals, which can be divided into actionable and measurable steps or stages, phased over time. The behaviour of children and adolescents needs to be clearly understood as distinct from adult behaviour and this will require good understanding of child and adolescent development. It will also require exploration of the young person in today's society with the current influences across the lifespan: for example, school, peer pressure, family beliefs and values and the media, which continue to have a powerful influence on the behaviour of young people.

3. **'Intervention mix' and 'marketing mix'**

   Using a range (or 'mix') of different interventions or methods to achieve a particular behavioural goal. When used at the strategic level this is commonly referred to as the 'intervention mix', and when used operationally it is described as the 'marketing mix' or 'social marketing mix'. A mix of interventions have proved to be successful with young people, in school and community: using advertising, providing listening services via mobile phones and internet sites, as well as accessible face-to-face services. Children and young people with different learning styles will need this mix of interventions in order to effectively target diverse needs.

4. **Audience segmentation**

   Clarity of audience focus using 'audience segmentation' to target effectively. Recognition here of the particular needs of a young audience in order to target effectively will be important.

5. **'Exchange'**

   Use and application of the 'exchange concept' – understanding what is being expected of 'the customer', the 'real cost to them'. This is a key area when considering young people. The drivers for young people to either change their health behaviour or prevent poor health choices will be very different from the decisions made by adults.

6. **'Competition'**

   Use and application of the 'competition concept' – understanding factors that impact on the customer and that compete for their attention and time. There are a number of competing 'pleasures' for a young person as they grow up, and social marketing in this context will have to consider how health messages can compete against the stronger influences of more unhealthy behaviours which are entrenched in adolescent behaviour, such as drugs, alcohol or smoking.

Increasingly, across government, the focus is on developing policy that is based on a sound understanding of the citizen, their lives and the communities they are part of. This is sometimes described as being *citizen-centric* (or alternatively *customer-centric* or *consumer-centric*), ensuring that policy is really driven by people's needs, wants and aspirations.

It is here that a social marketing perspective can directly contribute real insights and value. The core central feature of social marketing is its focus on understanding the *citizen/customer/consumer* and developing a profound insight into their lives ,thus avoiding professional assumptions about what they want, need, or think. Social marketers can check out and pre-test developing insights.

Part of the process in social marketing is establishing the 'exchange' potential. This involves making the offer to the customer or client and then working out the cost to them. This means understanding what the person has to give in order to get the proposed benefit; this might be time, effort, money, social consequences, and loss of pleasure. The practitioner involved has to understand how the offer can be enhanced to maximise the benefits, while working to minimise potential or actual blocks or barriers to it.

The health promoter needs to recognise that whatever is being 'offered' will always face competition, both external and internal; this might be the power of pleasure, habit or addiction. The strategy can include direct counter-messages and competing offers or simply competition for the time and attention of the same target customer/audience. The aim is about getting the right balance between benefit to the customer/consumer versus cost to customer/consumer. To take an example of where the social marketing model has been applied one could look at a case study from *Health Challenge England – Next Steps for Choosing Health* (DH, 2008).

Positive action: obesity prevention social marketing programme

The underlying approach to this programme is to identify a small number of key attitudinal and behavioural influences within childhood obesity and align as many resources as possible against these focus points to deliver positive changes. This will be achieved through developing a common strategy with partners based on these influences. In order to achieve this, the team at the Department of Health worked with stakeholders to bring together academic and market research from across government, the academic community, non-government organisations and the commercial sector to identify the key focus areas:

- Parents are unable to assess their personal/family weight status and/or do not appreciate the associated risks of being overweight and the connection with their day-to-day behaviours.
- Parents are not embracing healthy eating and active lifestyles because they are, or are perceived to be, abnormal or 'too challenging'.
- The level and nature of parental influence over the food habits of their children.
- Parents are subject to pressures that act to increase sedentary behaviour and discourage everyday activity.

Within each of these focus areas the specific behaviours, their drivers and the barriers to change have been identified. One successful strategy that has been developed to deal with these issues has been the MEND (Mind, Exercise, Nutrition, Do it!) project (Sacher *et al.*, 2007) (see Chapter 5). This is run on 230 sites in the UK and offers young people aged seven to thirteen the opportunity to get involved with sport and physical activities and gives their families advice and information about healthy eating and improving confidence and self-esteem.

MEND aims to provide families with the life skills to help children lead healthy, active lifestyles, preventing weight gain in a society overloaded by fast foods and technology, which encourage a sedentary lifestyle. Those taking part in the programme are given professional support and advice in developing healthy attitudes and behaviours around food and physical activity. Thanks to the Big Lottery funding, the programme is provided free of charge to participating families.

To apply the social marketing model to this initiative one can see that there is an exchange going on here between the health care professionals and the children with their families. The health care professionals are 'selling' the idea that taking part in exercise and gaining knowledge about what constitutes a healthy diet can be fun and may result in weight loss. It also encourages families to engage in activities together; therefore what the programme is selling is a positive message that the MEND programme is enjoyable and may bring some positive health benefits.

The other important aspect is the regular contact with the health promoters running the course who offer support and encouragement to the families so that they are not expected to get on with it on their own. This may lead to longer term benefits.

Conclusion

There are many health challenges facing young people today and community and school nurses are ideally placed to help families deal with these. However, health care professionals will need a good understanding of health promotion and its theory to enable them to construct interventions that will achieve the effect needed. This chapter has offered a range of models for consideration and a discussion of how they work in practice. There are many more examples of health promotion models than those discussed in this chapter. However, those presented here indicate that there are those that explain individual behaviour and how one can change behaviour. As part of the whole picture of health promotion explanations for individual behaviour and models which emphasise the importance of understanding the influences on individual behaviour are important. It is also important to understand which stage individuals are at when you are attempting to encourage them to take positive steps to improve their health chances.

Models that consider health promotion at the community level pay attention to the influence of the socio-economic and physical environments on health and how health promotion can take these into account. The models presented in this chapter show that health promotion is made up of many activities that go beyond health education and behaviour change. What is clear is that models have the potential to help health care professionals choose from a range of activities aimed at improving the health of individuals and communities. They also encourage us to plan our health promotion so that we can approach particular issues from a range of perspectives, thus increasing our chances of success.

References

Bandura, A. (2000) Cultivate self efficacy for personal and organisational effectiveness In: *The Blackwell Handbook of Principles of Organisational Behaviour* (ed. E. A. Locks). Blackwell, Oxford.

Beattie, A. (1991) Knowledge and control in health promotion: a test case for social policy and social theory. In *The Sociology of the Health Service* (eds. J. Gabe, M. Calnan and M. Bury). Routledge, London.

Bunton, R. and MacDonald, G. (2002) *Health Promotion: Disciplines, Diversity and Developments*, 2nd edn. Routledge, London.

British Medical Association (2008) *Measles, Mumps and Rubella (MMR) vaccine.* http://www.bma.org.uk/ap.nsf/Content/measlesmrvaccine; accessed 23 February 2008.

Davies, M. and MacDowall, W. (2006) *Health Promotion Theory*. Open University Press, Maidenhead.

Department for Education and Skills (1999) *National Healthy Schools Standard.* DfES, London.

Department of Health (2004a) *Immunisation Capital Catch Up Campaign.* Stationery Office, London.

Department of Health (2004b) *Choosing Health: Making Healthier Choices Easier.* DH, London.

Department of Health (2006) *Childhood Immunisations.* DH, London.

Department of Health (2008) *Health Challenge England – Next Steps for Choosing Health.* DH, London.

Downie, R. S., Tanahill, C. and Tannahill, A. (1996) *Health Promotion Models and Values*, 2nd edn. Open University Press, Oxford.

Ewles, L. and Simnett, I. (2003) *Promoting Health: a Practical Guide.* Scutari Press, London.

Hastings, G. and Haywood, A. (2002) Social marketing and communication in health promotion. *Health Promotion International*, **6**(2), 135–45.

Housten, F. S. and Gassenheimer, G. B. (1987) Marketing and Exchange. *Journal of Marketing*, **51**, 3–18.

Ledwith, M. (2005*) Community Development: a Critical Approach*. The Policy Press, Bristol.

National Social Marketing Centre for Excellence (2005) *Social Marketing Pocket Guide*. National Social Marketing Centre for Excellence, London.

Nutbeam, D. (2003) The health promoting school: closing the gap between theory and practice *Health Promotion International*, **7**(3), 151–3.

Nutbeam, D. and Harris, E. (2004) *Theory in A Nutshell: A Practical Guide to Health Promotion Theory*, NSW McGraw-Hill, Sydney.

Prochaska, J. O., DiClemente, C. C. and Norcross, J. C. (1992) In search of how people change: applications to addictive behaviours. *American Psychologist*, **47**, 1102–14.

Sacher, P., Chadwick, P., Kolotourou, M., Cole, T. J., Lawson, M. and Singhal, A. (2007) The MEND RCT: effectiveness on health outcomes in obese children. *International Journal of Obesity*, **31**(suppl. 1), S12.

Tones, K. and Tilford, S. (2001) *Health Promotion: Effectiveness, Efficiency and Equity*, 3rd edn. Nelson Thorne, Cheltenham.

Wakefield, A. J., Murch, S. H., Anthony, A., *et al.* (1998) Ileal-lymphoid-nodular hyperplasia, non-specific colitis, and pervasive developmental disorder in children. *Lancet*, **351** (9103), 637–41.

Wanless, D. (2004) *Good Health for the Whole Population: Final Report*, February 2004. DH, London.

World Health Organization (2008) *Immunizations, Vaccines and Biologicals.* http://www.who.int/immunization/en/; Accessed 23 February 2008.

CHAPTER 5

Contributing to personal, social and health education programmes

Elaine Tabony

Key themes

- Working within the curriculum
- Teaching strategies
- Education policy
- Personal, social, health education (PSHE) programmes – tackling key public health priorities

Introduction

Personal, social and health education (PSHE) and citizenship provide planned social and emotional support to children and young people, enabling a sense of identity and ability to make informed choices (Bird *et al.*, 2003; Blake, 2006). This chapter examines the relationship between policy and implementation, impact on learning and contribution to positive health outcomes for young people. Central to policy is the Children's National Service Framework, which has driven a cultural shift towards children and family services that improves life chances. Key drivers for this policy included the death of Victoria Climbié in February 2000. Victoria came into contact with health, police and social care services, but all failed to recognise abuse or prevent her death (Laming, 2003). In January 2002, a public inquiry report into the deaths of children following heart surgery at Bristol led to a commitment by the Department of Health to design a service to meet the needs of children that is safe and of highest quality. Policy emerged as *Every Child Matters: Change for Children (*Department of Health [DH]/Department for Education and Skills [DfES], 2004), setting a vision to support young people to realise five outcomes. *Every Child Matters: Change for Children* (DH/DfES, 2004) has 26 Public Service Agreement (PSA) targets and 13 other key indicators. In October 2004, the *Healthy Living Blueprint* for schools was launched, providing a platform for the *National Healthy Living Standard* (DfES, 2004). To support achievement of National Healthy School Status a plethora of policies over the last ten years have been published (Department for Education and Employment [DfEE], 1999; DH, 1999; DfEE, 2000; DH, 2001; DH/DfES, 2004; DfES, 2004; DfES, 2005). Schools are required to take a whole school approach to PSHE to include Sex and Relationships (SRE) and drug education, healthy eating, physical activity, emotional health and well-being (including bullying). Revision and update of the National Healthy Schools Programme (NHSP) standards provides an essential guide for schools to develop an effective PSHE programme (Ofsted, 2007).

Recent publications warn that this generation of children are likely to die before their parents due to lifestyle changes (DH, 2006; Aynsley-Green, 2007; Brill, 2007). To reverse trends, PSHE and development of Healthy Schools is central to aid a shift toward healthier living and positive lifestyle changes. To enhance the sustainability of positive life change, peer support programmes are evidenced as positive, effective methods of delivering PSHE. Enabling health, independence and well-being starts in childhood (DH, 2006).

Working within the curriculum – building success

Schools provide spiritual, moral, social and cultural support reflected through the school ethos positively affecting the curriculum outcomes for Personal, Social and Health Education (PSHE) (Bird *et al.*, 2003; DfES, 2005; Blake, 2006). Physical and emotional health impact on learning, yet schools vary in how they tackle these issues (Healey, 2002). Ofsted inspections report a failure of some schools to allow pupils to explore issues effectively in curriculum PSHE. Teaching time for PSHE is often restricted due to curriculum demands, with emphasis placed on subject knowledge and understanding of a narrow PSHE curriculum (DfES, 2005). Mental health and well-being, parenting education and financial awareness education are frequently neglected areas of the PSHE curriculum. Numerous schools pass PSHE responsibilities to form tutors causing a lack of clarity in their roles, often leading teachers towards favouring target setting and monitoring pupil progress. Schools where 'specialist teams' of teachers with additional subject knowledge deliver PSHE create the richest learning environment for effective exploration of PSHE (Ofsted, 2005a).

PSHE and Citizenship lie at the core of the National Curriculum (Bird *et al.*, 2003), reflecting the World Health Organization (WHO) (WHO, 1998) and European Union 'Health for All Targets' where Target 7 states that schools are particularly important settings in which programmes can be geared to encourage high self-esteem. Furthermore, all children should be supported to reach their full physical, mental and social potential. All professionals are obliged by law to support children to achieve the five outcomes proposed in the Outcomes Framework (The Children Act [DH], 2004a).

Standards are set by the Qualifications and Curriculum Authority (QCA) to ensure that the foundation blocks are laid to build upon throughout each key stage of learning. The Qualifications and Curriculum Authority offers best practice guidelines for all Key Stages with outcome expectations at completion of each Key Stage. The QCA is a non-departmental public body sponsored by the DfES that combines regulation of the public examination system and develops the national curriculum and the national qualification framework. The Qualifications and Curriculum Authority (QCA, 2000) advocates a whole-school approach to PSHE and Citizenship to ensure that classroom learning extends throughout the school. Staff training and development to facilitate a positive and nurturing ethos within all areas of the school empowers staff to foster a sense of community (Bird *et al.*, 2003; Blake, 2006). In order to meet National Healthy School Standards (NHSS) and Continuing Professional Development (CPD) teachers and community nurses will promote age-appropriate knowledge, skills and understanding. The key responsibility will be to develop pupil confidence and responsibility and make the most of their abilities. In order to succeed in a whole school approach, QCA advocates a clear policy link between PSHE and citizenship throughout relevant policies such as anti-bullying policy and child protection. Subject managers and teachers should be specifically responsible for PSHE and citizenship and a lead governor identified to assist in developing and managing process and implementation of PSHE and Citizenship (Bird *et al.*, 2003; Blake 2006).

The National PSHE Continuing Professional Development Programme

Nationally, over four phases of delivery, 8,000 teachers and community nurses have completed certification to enhance their professional development (DfES, 2004; Ofsted, 2007). Programme aims include improving confidence and competence in delivering PSHE, raising quality of teaching, learning and planning of PSHE. Teachers and community nurses follow the same standards for Dimension A: *The context and core skills of supporting teaching and learning in PSHE* and Dimension B: *Knowledge and understanding and their application to SRE*. Recognition of health professional input to PSHE is reflected in Standards Dimension C: *Community Nurses' unique contribution to PSHE: Contribution to partnership working and Health advice and support*. As part of wider Government initiatives such as the Teenage Pregnancy Strategy (Social Exclusion Unit [SEU], 1999), programme aims will raise standards, improve quality of PSHE through National Assessment and improve competence and confidence in PSHE delivery (DfEE, 2003; Ofsted, 2007).

Partnership between health and education is crucial in the development of the PSHE CPD. The role of the school nurse complements the teacher's role rather than replaces it (De Bell and Jackson, 2000; DH, 2001; DH/DfES, 2006; DH, 2006). Schools are required to plan, manage, deliver and evaluate their PSHE programme. The unique contribution of the community nurse envelops caseload knowledge, including children and young people not in mainstream school, linking local and national targets and involvement in policy review. Health advice and support includes providing one-to-one information to help young people manage their own health through assessment and agreed planning with the young person. Clear identification of the community nurse role in child protection is required. School nurses act as health advisors to parents, carers, teachers and others, particularly in relation to access to local health services (De Bell and Jackson, 2000; DH, 2001; Bailey *et al.*, 2007). The standards are reflected in recent government policies (SEU, 1999; DH, 2001; DH/DfES, 2004; DH, 2006).

Teaching strategies

Steady improvement in quality of teaching and learning in PSHE has been evidenced over the past five years (Ofsted, 2007). Disparity occurs in both primary and secondary school teaching of PSHE where there is lack of discussion and reflection time for pupils to debate constructively. Successful lessons occur where teachers have deep insight into the subject and have planned in partnership, particularly in Sex and Relationships Education (SRE). Variations in quality of teaching are prevalent where form tutors with only general subject knowledge teach PSHE. Session delivery can be enhanced through senior leadership ensuring that all teachers are supported through a subject coordinator to be fully involved in lesson planning (Ofsted, 2005b, 2006, 2007). Schools supporting form tutor delivery of PSHE suggest that the relationship level of pupil and tutor enhances personal and social development. Ofsted (2007) argue that the change of relationship and lack of subject knowledge impedes learning through form teachers' personal inhibitions on certain subjects, lack of understanding of suitable teaching methods, and negative or embarrassed reactions. Specialist teams teaching PSHE use wide-ranging teaching strategies, including paired work, small group discussion, games and role-play.

Developing effective delivery of PSHE requires the engagement of key partners in policy development, professional and practice (curriculum) development (Bird *et al.*, 2003; Ofsted, 2005a; Blake, 2006). Partners include pupil and parent involvement, including surveys and discussion. Additionally, school nurse, wider community, religious leaders, 'Healthy Schools' coordinators and national organisations working as a task group aid in a needs assessment-led curriculum development of PSHE. Central to policy development is the need to assess the knowledge gained. A minority of schools attempt to assess knowledge and understanding of PSHE. Ofsted (2007) generally find this area weak, particularly observing for change of attitude and developing skills. The new schools inspection framework strengthens the role of PSHE and advice from QCA supports schools in PSHE impact assessment (Ofsted, 2007).

Professional development of teachers should cover aspects relating to law, skills and confidence, confidentiality and peer review. Furthermore, staff may require emotional support and reflective opportunities (Bird *et al.*, 2003; Blake, 2006). Curriculum development needs to be broad, maximising the unique contributions that can be made by those in other disciplines, particularly health professionals. Commitment to joined-up approaches should be shared by all professionals (DH, 2004b), cementing links across health, education and voluntary services.

Importance is placed on teachers ensuring that PSHE lessons use a variety of learning strategies, for example involving pupils in discussion or role-play. The classroom climate needs to foster security in pupils expressing feelings and respect for fellow pupil attitudes and beliefs (Ofsted, 2005a, 2007). Sensitive issues such as homophobic bullying and lack of knowledge of HIV and AIDS should be addressed. Advice and support for professionals is available through the Sex Education Forum on line as well as regular training sessions in sensitive subject areas. Ofsted (2007) report sensitivity of subjects creates a challenge for teachers who do not always stimulate a challenge to prejudice.

Assessment of PSHE key issues is often absent from lessons and reports to parents. Where assessment has been addressed good practice includes gathering evidence from pupil comments, discussion, observation and written reflection by pupils (Ofsted, 2007). Assessment aids include attainment outcomes developed by the QCA for knowledge skills and understanding in PSHE at the end of each key stage of learning (QCA, 2007).

Confidentiality for teachers and nurses varies according to the situation. Health professionals involved in PSHE programme delivery follow school policy in classroom situations and their own professional code of conduct in one-to-one situations (DfEE, 2000; Ofsted, 2007). Teachers are not required by law to break confidentiality unless child protection issues apply (Ofsted,

2007). Schools should have a confidentiality policy and staff aware of its content and procedure. Awareness of the *Common Assessment Framework* and Safeguarding policy is mandatory for all staff.

Education policy

A 'Healthy School' demonstrates a whole school approach, involving representatives of the entire school community to develop PSHE for these subjects: Sex and Relationships Education (SRE) and Drug education (including alcohol, tobacco and volatile substance abuse); Healthy eating, physical activity and emotional health and well-being (including bullying) (Ofsted 2005b). A 'Healthy School' plans PSHE following DfES and Qualifications and Curriculum Authority (QCA) guidance and involves external agencies in developing PSHE. Developing a whole school approach to PSHE within the National Healthy School Programme involves 10 core principles explored for each of the four key themes (Health Development Agency [HDA], 2006):

- Leadership, management, and managing change
- Policy development, e.g. SRE, drug education
- Curriculum planning and resourcing, including working with external agencies
- Teaching and learning
- School culture and environment
- Giving pupil's a voice
- Provision of pupil's support services
- Staff professional development needs
- Health and welfare partnerships with parents, carers and local communities
- Assessing, recording and reporting pupil achievements

Subsequent to the *Every Child Matters* (ECM) agenda, establishing a baseline for good practice in PSHE has been undertaken by Ofsted inspection and published as 'Healthy schools, healthy children?'. Survey inclusion of 18 schools (10 primary, 6 secondary and 2 special schools) was generated by NHSP accreditation prior to the rigorous new criteria (Ofsted, 2006). Based on the 'Healthy Living Blueprint for Schools' (DfES, 2004), schools were required to evidence progress with the five outcomes as shown in Table 5.1.

The National Healthy Schools Programme (NHSP) builds on the previous National Healthy Schools Standard (NHSS) with the inclusion of the Con-

Table 5.1 Healthy Living Blueprint for Schools (DfES, 2004).

Objective 1
Promoting a school ethos and environment which encourage a healthy lifestyle

Objective 2
Using the full capacity and flexibility of the curriculum to achieve a healthy lifestyle

Objective 3
Ensuring that food and drink are available across the school day
Reinforce the healthy lifestyle message

Objective 4
Providing high-quality physical education and school sport and promoting physical activity

Objective 5
Promoting an understanding of the full range of issues and behaviours which impact on lifelong health

tinuing Professional Development (CPD) programme for both Teachers and Community Nurses. The aims of the NHSP are to support children and young people in developing healthy behaviours; help raise pupil achievement; to help to reduce health inequalities; and promote social inclusion. For schools to receive National Healthy School Status a rigorous assessment process ensues where schools are required to achieve competence in all four themes before being awarded this recognition.

Key findings showed a link between positive impact on learning and strong commitment to the NHSP to improve pupil and staff health and well-being. PSHE played an important part in the improvement yet the assessment guidance from QCA was rarely used (Ofsted, 2006). DfES and DH recommendations promote schools to make a positive contribution to pupil's health through NHSP. Local authorities are urged to improve the quality of meals not prepared on school premises. The cornerstone of health promotion within the NHSP is parent and pupil involvement in promoting healthier lifestyles. Schools are required by Ofsted to submit Self Evaluation Forms (SEF) over a three-year cycle. demonstrating the links to ECM outcomes and School Improvement. Forms differ from the Children's Centre SEF submitted on an annual basis to the Local Authority, which act as an annual management performance exercise.

Barriers to improving PSHE impact directly on pupils. For example, if transition to secondary school has not been effectively managed regarding the emotional demands on a child, pupils take longer to settle, or if liaison is minimal regarding previous learning, pupils fail to engage due to repeat of earlier work (Ofsted, 2006). The environment has a similar effect; for example, poor dining facilities, limited menu choice or long dinner queue will affect pupils' willingness to eat in school canteens (Ofsted, 2006).

The five outcomes outlined in *Change for Children – Every Child Matters* (ECM) (DH/DfES, 2004) are be healthy; stay safe; enjoy and achieve; make a positive contribution; and achieve economic well-being. Children and young people will be supported to gain those outcomes, as the NHS is central to achieving these targets. NHS staff will work towards developing Children's Trusts as cooperatives negotiating, delivering and commissioning education and social care. Information-sharing policies as part of the Common Assessment Framework will bridge all services. Commencing in the most deprived areas, access to services is viewed as paramount. Local authorities will support 'healthy schools' to develop into 'extended schools' creating health and social care networks for the wider community (DH/DfES, 2004). Part of this agenda is the establishment of Children's Centres offering early years education, parental and health support.

School nursing and PSHE

The child-centred public health approach identifies school nurses as key health professionals in building relationships to work with individuals, groups and communities to identify and meet the health needs of the school age population (DH, 2006). Involvement of school nurses in public health spreads from community level programmes, through whole school and community group work, to working with individuals (DH/DfES, 2006). School nurses are ideally placed to help reduce health inequalities and support access to services for those in most need (De Bell and Jackson, 2000; DH, 2006).

The Chief Nursing Officer (CNO) Review (DH, 2004) defined the school nurse role as working with children, young people, parents and carers, teaching staff, and others by providing general information, advice and support about health issues. School nurses would support learning about risk management and making healthy choices. School nurses are seen as key contributors to the Healthy Schools Programme through support for children to develop healthy behaviours and raise their achievement, and helping to reduce inequalities and promote social inclusion. Viewed as a valuable resource, the CNO will work with School Nurse leaders and the DfES to modernise and promote the service (DfES/DH, 2006).

An example of how school nursing strives toward meeting health priorities in Hillingdon Primary Care Trust is shown in Table 5.2. The table is an

Table 5.2 School nursing in Hillingdon 2007 and Every Child Matters (adapted from *Every Child Matters: Change for Children 2004*).

Be healthy	Stay safe	Enjoy and achieve	Make a positive contribution	Achieve economic well-being
Physical health MEND project, health assessments; PSHE CPD programme; health assessments and health screening	**Safe from maltreatment, neglect, violence, sexual exploitation** Child protection support; partnerships with domestic violence support groups	**Ready for school** New to school parent talks; Health Visitor to School Nurse handover for vulnerable families	**Engage in decision making and support the community and environment** School Council partnership working	**Engage in education, employment, or training on leaving school** Vulnerable children assessment/ support
Mentally and emotionally Seasons for Growth – Grief education – Tier 2 psycho-social intervention – Suicide prevention; drop-ins, CAMHS joint work; vulnerable children; assessment/support	**Safe from accidental injury and death** Junior Citizenship Partnership Project – offered to all 10/11 year olds – accidents, medicine safety, smoking, alcohol, substance abuse; PSHE partnership working in schools	**Attend and enjoy school** Partnership working; Educational Welfare Officer joint work; one-to-one working; health drop-ins; Seasons for Growth grief education	**Engage in law abiding and positive behaviour out of school** Self-esteem, one-to-ones, school health drop-in; Youth Inclusion Support Programme (YISP) attendance meetings; liaison with community police officers	**Ready for employment** Vulnerable children work; school health drop-in; partnership working with Connexions advisors
Sexually Healthy PSHE CPD certificate; teenage pregnancy strategy; access to services talks in school; STI and teenage pregnancy; drop-ins	**Safe from bullying and discrimination** Drop-in; one-to-one; peer support; partnership in developing school policies	**Achieve stretching national educational standards <11** Ensuring ability to access education; health assessments; audio/vision screening	**Develop positive relationships and choose not to bully or discriminate** Support in special schools; advocacy of the school-age child	**Live in decent homes and sustainable communities** Home visits; community partnerships; HAVS, children's fund; multi-agency working
Healthy lifestyles PSHE; MEND programme; smoking, drugs and alcohol – junior citizenship	**Safe from crime and anti-social behaviour in and out of school** Multi-disciplinary team partnership working; vulnerable children working – care plans	**Achieve personal, social development and enjoy recreation** One-to-one support; school health drop-in; MEND programme	**Develop self-confidence and successfully deal with life changes and challenges** Seasons for Growth grief education; school health; drop-in/one-to-one support	**Access to transport and material goods** Multi-Disciplinary team partnership work in areas of deprivation
Choose not to take illegal drugs Junior citizenship programme; PSHE partnership lesson/ working	**Have security stability and are cared for** Child protection and children in care health assessment clinics; school health assessments	**Achieve stretching national educational standards >11** Case load to 19 years; 6th form PSHE; drop-in	**Develop enterprising behaviour** Promoting self-esteem – one-to-one/peer support; Seasons for Growth Grief education	**Live in households free from low income** Working in partnership with families on low income

example of how policies are implemented and transferred into practice. The NSF plays a pivotal delivery role in the 'Be Healthy' aspect of ECM supported by further documents linking the first five standards to all children and young people, standards 6 to 10 for those with complex needs and standard 11 to Midwifery services. Key principles followed in the public health white paper *Choosing Health – Making Healthy Choices Easier* drew services to tackle inequalities through education, health and social care, shortly followed by the *Children Bill* (2004) and *Supporting Local Delivery* (HM Treasury, 2004; DfES/DH, 2004c).

PSHE courses – tackling key public health priorities

Health education is a core theme of PSHE in schools where promoting a healthier lifestyle embeds the curriculum. Schools that identify the link between physical and emotional well-being and learning and achieving are most effective in supporting pupils to achieve their potential. Self-esteem, positive behaviours, nourishment and keeping safe need to be well coordinated and reinforced for pupils to realise links as part of a healthy lifestyle (Ofsted, 2005a,b, 2007). The term 'Health Education' popular in the 1970s has been described as narrow and individualistic, with a sense of 'victim blaming' (Ewles and Simnett, 2004; Naidoo and Wills, 2005). 'Health Promotion', popular since the 1980s covers the broader issues of empowerment and control to improve health. The focus of Public Health takes a societal approach to preventing disease, prolonging life and promoting health. Health Education Programmes are health promotion activities supporting people to explore an aspect of health enabling voluntary behaviour change and improving self-esteem (Ewles and Simnett, 2004). The Public Health approach aims to improve the health of populations. Key issues for public health are the steep rise in childhood obesity, mental health of young people and sexual health, including teenage pregnancy. Health and education workers may work with individuals to promote health or undertake health education programmes involving peer support to tackle these issues.

Tackling childhood obesity

Childhood obesity has risen dramatically over the past three decades, often linked to deprivation in western society (Lobstein *et al.*, 2004; Jotangia *et al.*, 2006; Wang and Lobstein, 2006; Doak *et al.*, 2006). Tackling childhood obesity is a key Public Service Agreement (PSA) target and key priority for school nursing (DfES/DH, 2005; NICE, 2006; DH, 2006). Three government departments; the Department of Health (DH), Department for Education and Skills (DfES) and Department for Culture Media and Sport (DCMS) share the PSA target.

One support programme tackling childhood obesity is known as MEND. (Mind, Exercise, Nutrition, Do it!). Written by Paul Sacher, specialist paediatric dietician and Paul Chadwick, doctor of clinical psychology, the programme is a community-based multidisciplinary treatment and prevention programme for obese and overweight children and their families. A Randomised Controlled Trial (RCT) has been completed; results were presented at the European Congress of Obesity in 2007 (Sacher *et al.*, 2007) and will be published. MEND is a lifestyle behaviour change programme accessed by the family at a time they feel ready to make positive changes.

Health promoters considering use of 'stage models' to aid recognition of a families readiness to change could consider using the Transtheoretical Model (Prochaska *et al.*, 1992) or Precaution Adoption Process Model (Weinstein, 1988). Rutter and Quine (2005) debate whether one passes through stages within theoretical models or through random points on a continuum.

A joint initiative led by Hillingdon Primary Care Trust (PCT) involving partnership between DfES and DCMS and part of a PSHE programme has been the introduction of the MEND programme. The age range for group work is 7–13 years old. Outcomes of the local pilot study mirrored results previously published by the MEND research team at the University College London Institute of Child Health and Great Ormond Street Hospital for Sick Children (Sacher, 2005; Sacher *et al.*, 2005a,b, 2006a,b, 2007). The results included reduced waist circumference, improved cardiovascular fitness and increased self-esteem.

As a peer support initiative, MEND is an 18 session, nine-week programme for children and their families to attend (Table 5.3). Parents attend twice a week with their child for two-hour sessions. The first hour involves an interactive workshop session that alternates between nutrition education and behaviour change sessions largely aimed at parents. The second hour comprises a multi-skills exercise session for the children. Thorough evaluation is conducted pre- and post-Programme to determine effectiveness of this national standardised child obesity programme.

MEND affords the opportunity for different professionals to work in partnership in order to achieve positive outcomes. Involvement of the School Nursing Service provides a health link and an opportunity to address any emotional health issues that may have arisen due to bullying or poor self-esteem at the child's school.

Table 5.3 MEND programme content (adapted from *MEND Programme Manual, Version 5*, Sacher and Chadwick, 2007).

Mind	Exercise	Nutrition
Eight sessions designed to improve self-esteem and behaviour change. These sessions support changes in children's habits around eating and exercising using e.g. goals and reward setting, triggers and modelling.	Eighteen sessions of multi-skills, graded, non-competitive group based exercise on land or water designed to be inclusive. Activities encourage team building, increased balance, agility and co-ordination and improve fitness.	Eight sessions designed to empower families by enabling them to make educated choices around nutrition. Sessions include unrefined carbohydrates, label reading, cooking, fats and sugars, eating out and special occasions as well a supermarket tour. No diet is recommended.

Mental health and psychological well-being

Mental health problems are prevalent in schools with around 10% of children or young people requiring professional help. Links have been identified between untreated childhood mental health problems and academic failure, offending behaviour and substance misuse (DH, 2006). Programmes that address self-esteem issues and mental ill health are advocated as a PSA target (DH, 2004a,b). Factors that affect mental health problems in young people are outlined in Table 5.4.

Seasons for Growth is a Grief Education Peer Support Programme addressing issues concerning loss and change. In health education terms the Seasons for Growth programme crosses Tier 1 and Tier 2 of the Child and Adolescent Mental Health Service (CAMHS) four-tier framework through opportunity to promote mental health and prevent mental health problems (DH/DfEE, 1995; Audit Commission, 1999). It is a psychosocial intervention to support children and young people to increase skills to cope, improve communication and problem solving. Seasons for Growth is a nine session programme, 50 minutes per session, written at five different levels for children and young people to access at an appropriate level of understanding. Following Commonwealth Government of Australia Evaluation (Muller and Wraith, 1999), parents and teaching staff had noted significant improvement in behaviour and concentration and requested an adult programme to meet parent needs. Further evaluation in 2005 showed statistically significant findings in increasing optimism and

Table 5.4 Risk Factors for mental health problems in young people (adapted from Audit Commission, 1999; Pearse and Holmes, 1994).

Child risk factors	Family risk factors	Environmental risk factors
Genetic influences	Overt parental conflict	Homelessness
Learning disability and low IQ	Inconsistent or unclear discipline	Socio-economic disad-vantge
Developmental delay	Family breakdown	Disaster
Communication issues	Hostile and rejecting relationships	Discrimination
Difficult temperament	Failure to adapt to a child's developmental needs	Other significant life events
Academic failure	Abuse	
Chronic physical illness	Parental criminality, alcoholism and person-ality disorder	
Low self-esteem	Death and loss – includ-ing friendships	
	Parental psychiatric illness	

problem solving, breaking down isolation, enhancing self-esteem, awakening hope and increasing resilience (Frydenberg and Muller, 2005).

Over 90,000 children and young people across 7 countries have partici-pated in the programme since it was written by Dr Anne Graham in 1996. The theoretical framework is found in the work of J. William Worden's 'tasks of grief' (Worden, 1995) and adapted to educational settings distinct from a clinical setting. The programme does not offer counselling or therapy but offers an environment of mutual support facilitated by a 'Companion'. 'Tasks' underpinning the Seasons for Growth Grief Education programme is (Graham, 1996, 1998, 2002):

- The participants are supported to come to terms with the reality of their loss.
- Children and young people are given the opportunity to learn about the range of emotions that accompany grief and how each has experienced these in his/her own loss.
- The participants are provided with skills to assist in processing their grief.

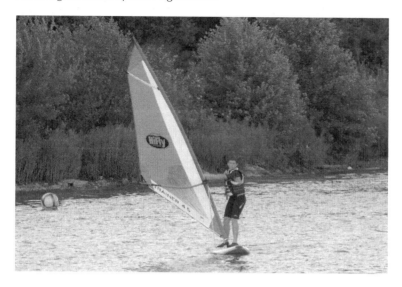

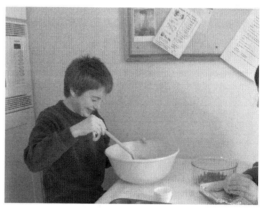

PSHE encourages young people to take physical exercise and to eat in a healthy way

- The participants are given the opportunity to explore ways of letting go and moving on.

Seasons for Growth 'normalises' the process of grief, enabling participants to gain knowledge and understand feelings and the effects of loss. The distinction between 'normal' grief work and where a person may be 'stuck' in grief is important to recognise. Appropriate referral to a clinical setting in CAMHS framework Tier 3 is advised if a person is 'stuck' in grief (Graham, 1996). Training as a facilitator or 'Companion' is available to all professionals in CAHMS Tier 1, including teachers, school surses and health visitors.

Sex and Relationships Education (SRE)

Significant changes in policies relating to Sex and Relationships Education policy have been advocated over the past twenty years. In 1988, Section 28 of the Local Government Act prohibited promoting homosexuality and acceptability as a pretended family relationship (Young, 2004). Fifteen years later in 2003 this clause was repealed. In 1996 the Education Act set out mandatory SRE elements in the National Curriculum Science Order to include teaching about Sexually Transmitted Infections, including HIV. Local programmes of SRE were introduced through the DfEE as the National Healthy School Standard in 1999, shortly followed by SRE guidance (DfEE, 2000).

SRE has emerged as highly significant in terms of PSHE as the UK has one of the highest teenage pregnancy rates in Western Europe. Reducing teenage pregnancy is a key health target. Jointly the DfES and DH PSA target aim is to reduce teenage pregnancy by 50% by 2010 (DH, 2004a). Teenage parents are less likely to complete education and more likely to be unemployed and live in social deprivation (DH, 2006). Sexually Transmitted Infections (STIs) are prevalent in women under 25 years old, with estimates of up to 10% of sexually active young people having chlamydia, a leading cause of infertility (DH, 2006).

Addressing the problem of sexual health is complex. Young (2004) suggests that the way young people feel generally impacts on high risk-taking behaviours. Risk taking could involve excessive drinking and drug use, as well as having unprotected sex. The introduction of the relationships element of SRE offers young people a chance to explore emotions, gender issues, promote discussion, value self and value choice (Ofsted, 2002a,b,c, 2004, 2005a,b).

The NHSP CPD programme assists young people to achieve these aims. Education and health partnerships are an integral part of promoting health in SRE. School nurses can ensure that young people have access to services and information about contraception, screening programmes, emergency contraception, pregnancy and abortion (Young and Arnold-Dean, 2004; Bailey *et al.*, 2007). Although schools play a key role in tackling the issue there are a number of factors that challenge public health outcomes. These include reaching young people who have disengaged from education, socio-economic factors, parental attitudes and beliefs, parental withdrawal from SRE lessons and absence through illness (Young, 2004).

Conclusion

A number of positive initiatives have emerged in considering best practice in PSHE. Cooperation between services is paramount, with equal value placed on what each service has to offer. Care must be taken to address health inequalities and meet the needs of a generation disadvantaged by poverty, conflicting media messages and lack of knowledge (SEU, Report 1999). Delivery of high-quality PSHE relies on appropriately trained staff in health and education. Standards set in NHSP CPD broadly achieve these aims.

References

Aynsley-Green, A. (2007) Children's commissioner says obesity is endangering lives of thousands of children and young people. http://www.childrenscommissioner. org/adult/news/news.cfm?id=1964; accessed 26 January 2007.

Audit Commission (1999) *Children in Mind: Child and Adolescent Mental Health Services.* Audit Commission, London.

Bailey, C., Gateshill, P., Griffiths, L. and Lowe, K. (2007) *DfES CPD Programme for Community Nurses.* Surrey, VT Education and Skills.

Bird, J., Blake, S., Frances, G. and Muttock, S. (2003) *A Whole-School Approach to Personal, Social Health Education.* National Children's Bureau (NCB), London.

Blake, S. (2006) *A Whole-School Approach to Personal, Social Health Education.* National Children's Bureau (NCB), London.

Brill, B. (2007) Child obesity more than a cosmetic problem. http://www.nctimes.com/ articles/2007/02/18/news/carlsbad/17_52_381_1; accessed 18 February 2007.

De Bell, D. and Jackson, P. (2000) *School Nursing within the Public Health Agenda: a Strategy for Practice.* CPHVA, QNI, RCN, London.

Department for Education and Employment (DfEE) (1999) *National Healthy School Standard.* DfEE, London.

Department for Education and Employment (DfEE) (2000) *Guidance: Sex and Relationship Education.* DfEE, Nottingham.

Department for Education and Employment (DfEE) (2003) *National Healthy School Standard.* DfEE, Nottingham.

Department for Education and Skills (2004) *Healthy Living Blueprint for Schools.* DfES, Nottingham.

Department for Education and Skills (2005) *Social and Emotional Aspects of Learning – Guidance Document (Primary National Strategy, DfES 1378).* DfES, London.

Department for Education and Skills/Department of Health (2004) *Every Child Matters: Change for Children.* DfES/DH, London.

Department for Education and Skills and Department of Health (2005) *National Healthy Schools Status: a Guide for Schools.* DH Publications, London.

Department for Health and Department for Education (1995) *A Handbook on Child and Adolescent Mental Health.* HMSO, London.

Department of Health (1999) *Saving Lives: Our Healthier Nation.* Stationery Office, London.

Department of Health (2001) *School Nurse Development Resource Pack.* Stationery Office, London.

Department of Health (2004a) *The Children Act.* DH, London.

Department of Health (2004b) *Choosing Health: Making Healthier Choices Easier.* Stationery Office, Norwich.

Department of Health (2004c) *NSF for Children, Young People and Maternity Services: Supporting Local Delivery.* DfES Publications, Nottingham.

Department of Health (2006) *Our Health, Our Care, Our Say: A New Direction for Community Services.* Stationery Office, London.

Department of Health (DH)/Department for Education and Skills (DfES) (2006) *School Nurse: Development Resource Pack. Specialist Community Public Health Nurse.* DfES/DH, Nottingham.

Doak, C. M., Visscher, T. L. S., Renders, M. and Seiddell, J. C. (2006) The prevention of overweight and obese children and adolescents: a review of intervention programmes. *Obesity Reviews,* **7**(1), 111–36.

Ewles, L. and Simnett, I. (2004) *Promoting Health: a Practical Guide,* 5th edn. Baillière Tindall, Edinburgh & London.

Frydenberg, E. and Muller, D. (2005) *Coping with Loss: An Evaluation of the Seasons for Growth Programme.* Mary McKillop Foundation, Melbourne.

Graham, A. P. (1996) *Seasons for Growth: Grief Education Programme.* Southern Cross University, New South Wales.

Graham, A. P. (1998) *Seasons for Growth: Grief Education Programme.* Southern Cross University, New South Wales.

Graham, A. P. (2002) *Seasons for Growth: Grief Education Programme.* Southern Cross University, New South Wales.

Healey, K. (2002) *A Good Place to Learn? What Young People Think Makes School Health.* Kings Fund, London.

Health Development Agency (HDA) (2005) *National Healthy Schools Programme: a Briefing for LEA School Improvement and Children's Service Officers, Specialist Agencies, Elected Members and School Communities.* NHSP, Yorkshire.

HM Treasury (2004) *Children Bill.* Stationery Office, London.

International Association for the Study of Obesity (IASO) (2007) *Childhood Obesity. Sydney Principle Consultation.* http://www.iotf.org/childhoodobesity.asp; accessed 27 January 2007.

Jotangia, D., Moody, A., Stamatakis, E. and Wardle, H. (2006) *Obesity Among Children Under 11.* National statistics. National Centre for Social Research (NatCen) Department of Epidemiology and Public Health at the Royal Free and University College Medical School, London.

Lobstein, T., Baur, L. and Uauy, R. (2004) IASO International Obesity Task Force (IOTF) Obesity in children and young people: a crisis in public health. *Obesity Reviews* (2004; 05), **1**(4), 104. Report to World Health Organization (WHO) (2004).

Laming, B. H. (2003) *The Victoria Climbié Inquiry, Report of an Inquiry by Lord Laming.* Stationery Office, London.

Muller, D. and Wraith, R. (1999) *An Evaluation of the Seasons for Growth Programme: Consolidated Report.* Irving Saulwick and Associates, Melbourne, Australia.

Naidoo, J. and Wills, J. (2005) *Public Health and Health Promotion. Developing Practice,* 2nd edn. Baillière Tindall, Edinburgh.

National Institute for Health and Clinical Excellence (NICE) (2006) *New NICE Guideline for Urgent Action to Stem the Rising Tide of Obesity in England and Wales.* NICE, London.

Ofsted (2002a) *Drug Education in Schools: an Update* (HMI 746). Ofsted, London.

Ofsted (2002b) *Sex and Relationships Education in Schools* (HMI 433). Ofsted, London.

Ofsted (2002c) *Sex and Relationships in Schools*. Ofsted, London.

Ofsted (2004) *Personal, Social and Health Education in Secondary Schools*. Ofsted, London.

Ofsted (2005a) *Drug Education in Schools* (HMI 2392). Ofsted, London.

Ofsted (2005b) *Personal, Social and Health Education in Schools* (HMI 2311). Ofsted, London.

Ofsted (2006) *Healthy Schools, Healthy Children? The Contribution of Education to Pupils' Health and Well-being*. Ofsted, London.

Ofsted (2007) *Time for Change? Personal, Social and Health Education*. Ofsted Reference 070049, London.

Pearse, J. and Holmes, S. (1994) 'Health Gain Investment Programme' Technical Review Document. *People with Mental Health problems (part four) – Child and Adolescent Mental Health*. NHS Executive Trent and Centre for Mental Health Services Development.

Prochaska, J. O., DiClemente, C. C. and Norcross, J. C. (1992) In search of how people change: applications to addictive behaviours. *American Psychologist*, **47**(9), 1102–14.

Qualifications and Curriculum Authority (QCA) (2000) *Personal, Social and Health Education and Citizenship at Key Stages 1 and 2: Initial Guidance for Schools*. QCA, London.

Rutter, D. and Quine, L. (2005) *Changing Health Behaviour*. Open University Press, Berkshire.

Sacher, P. M. (2005) Childhood obesity: consequences and control measures. *Journal of Family Health Care*. **15**(4), Spec. Suppl. 1, 4–5.

Sacher, P. M., Kolotourou, M., Chadwick, P., Singhal, A., Cole, T. J. and Lawson, M. (2002) Paediatric parenteral nutrition and nutrition support teams in the United Kingdom. *Proceedings of the Nutrition Society*, **2001**(60), 110A.

Sacher, P. M., Chadwick, P. and Hogan, L. (2002) The obesity epidemic. *Journal of Family Health Care*, **12**(4), 111.

Sacher, P. M., Kolotourou, M., Chadwick, P., Singhal, A., Cole, T. J. and Lawson, M. (2003) An integrated programme of nutrition, exercise and behavioural modification in a small group of obese 7–11 year old children. *Proceedings of the Nutrition Society*, **2003**(62), OCA/B,3A.

Sacher, P. M., Gray, C. and Lawson, M. (2005a) The MEND Programme is effective in reducing glycaemic load, total energy intake and waist circumference in a small group of obese 7–11 year old children. *Obesity Reviews*, **6**(suppl. 1), P410:121.

Sacher, P. M., Chadwick, P., Wells, J. C. K., Williams, J., Cole, T. J. and Lawson, M. (2005b) Assessing the acceptability and feasibility of the MEND Programme in a small group of obese 7–11 year old children. *Journal of Human Nutrition and Dietetics*, **18**, 3–5.

Sacher, P. M. and Chadwick, P. (2006) *Mend Programme Manual: Version 5*. MEND Central Ltd, London.

Sacher, P. M., Kolotourou, M., Chadwick, P., Singhal, A., Cole, T. J. and Lawson, M. (2006a) The MEND Programme: effectiveness on health outcomes in obese children. *Obesity Reviews*, **7**(2), 89.

Sacher, P. M., Kolotourou, M., Chadwick, P., Singhal, A., Cole, T. J. and Lawson, M. (2006b) Is the MEND Programme effective in improving health outcomes in obese children? *International Journal of Obesity*, **30**(2), S41.

Sacher, P. M. (2007) *The UK MEND Project Gets International Plaudits*. http://nationalobesityforum.org.uk/content/view/263/131/; accessed 7 January 2008.

Social Exclusion Unit (1999) *Teenage Pregnancy*. Home Office, London.

Wang, Y. and Lobstein, T. (2006) Worldwide trends in childhood overweight and obesity. *International Journal of Pediatric Obesity*, **1**, 11–25.

Wanless, D. (2003) *Securing Good Health for the Whole Population*. HM Treasury, London.

Weinstein, N. D. and Sandman, P. M. (1992) A model of precaution adoption process: evidence from home radon testing. *Health Psychology*, **11**(3), 170–80.

World Health Organization (1998) *Health 21 Strategy: The Introduction to Health for All Policy for the European Union*. WHO, Copenhagen.

Worden, J. W. (1995) *Grief Counselling and Grief Therapy: A Handbook for the Mental Health Practitioner*. Routledge, London.

Young, I. (2004) Exploring the role of schools in Sexual Health promotion. In: *Young People and Sexual Health: Individual, Social and Policy Contexts* (eds. E. Burtney and M. Duffy). Palgrave Macmillan, New York.

Young, B. and Arnold-Dean, W. (2004) *Personal, Social and Health Education (PSHE) Certification Programme for Community Nurses' Handbook*, rev. edn. Health Development Agency, Yorkshire.

Useful websites

M.E.N.D: http://www.nationalobesityforum.org.uk/content/blogcategory/23/176/

National Children's Bureau (NCB): http://www.ncb.org/

Seasons for Growth Grief Education Programme:

England and Wales: info@seasonsforgrowth.co.uk

Scotland: sfg@notredamecentre.org

CHAPTER 6

Parenting in the 21st century

Elizabeth Joy Power

Key themes

- Parenting challenges in the 21st century
- The challenges that both health care professionals and parents face in dealing with parenting in the 21st century
- The role of the Specialist Community Public Health Nurse in supporting parents

Parenting has always been an important issue, not just from a societal point of view, but also from an educational, emotional and economical position. Parenting in the 21st century is more pertinent now than it has ever been and is very high on the political agenda (DCSF, 2007). The quality of the relationship between parents and their children can have far-reaching consequences into adulthood. If there is a lack of positive parenting in infancy and beyond, the impact on the emotional, psychological and physical well-being of that person could have serious implications for their successful maturation into adulthood (Hardyment, 1995). In terms of government policy, the issue of parenting is no longer a concern only for those working within health. The repercussions of poor parenting now span across other government departments, including those responsible for education, crime and disorder, and social inequalities. The cost of sub-optimal parenting is high in terms of its impact on antisocial behaviour (Scott *et al.*, 2001a).

Parenting means different things to different people. It is often due to the diverse and complex interpretation of parenting that health care professionals find they have an onerous task on their hands. In its simplistic form the definition of parenting in the *Collins Pocket English Dictionary* (2000) cites the following: 'Parenting... the activity of bringing up children'.

Unfortunately, parenting is not just a case of "bringing up children". For successful parenting to take place, parents themselves need to be good role models (Sanders and Christensen, 1985). Parents include all those who carry out parenting duties, such as biological parents, single parents, gay and lesbian parents, step-parents, adoptive and foster parents, and other carers. As the world has evolved in terms of education, technology, transport and economical status, a break away from the traditional extended family has been seen. The extended family was stereotypically geographically compact with support mechanisms from both sides of the family readily available. In addition to this support mechanism, there were also very strong family morals and value systems. The role of parenting extended beyond the parents and was a shared responsibility amongst other family members. In today's society the nuclear family is presented as the norm, though for many adults and children this is not the case (Giddens, 2006). The nuclear family consists of two adults and, typically, two children, living in isolation from their immediate family. Many families live long distances apart and the economic demands of the 21st century require that both parents work (DCSF, 2007). The roles and opportunities for both men and women are continuously expanding and the ability to balance work with parental responsibilities can exert considerable pressure on those adults concerned, often to the detriment of their children. In addition, the constitution of the family is also shifting. The concept of the 'single parent' and the multi-dimensional aspect of many families as a result of divorce or separation is becoming the norm. The family dynamics within reconstituted families can significantly impact on the parent–child relationship (Wisensale, 1992).

Parents of the 21st century need to be confident with a strong sense of purpose and self-esteem (RCPCH, 2002). Optimal parenting requires unconditional love, warmth, affection, sensitivity, honesty and encouragement, with the creation of opportunities, as well as the ability to set firm but consistent age-appropriate boundaries (Gerhardt, 2004). Positive parenting embraces all of the above and facilitates the nurturing and growth of healthy infants through to childhood, adolescence and adulthood (Shaw and Stewart-Brown, 2004). Good parent–child relationships significantly reduce the risk to children of physical and mental disability (DH, 1999) as well as the adoption of unhealthy lifestyles, such as smoking, drinking and drug-taking (Stewart-Brown, 2000).

An absence of sensitive care from a consistent caregiver in the first two years of life and beyond can have dire consequences for a safe and cognitively smooth transition into adulthood (Shore, 1997). A lack of emotional warmth, security and positive discipline can result in severely disordered emotional and social development. This may exhibit itself in adolescence through to adulthood by means of anti-social, criminal and delinquent behaviour (Shore, 1997). The likelihood of successful interpersonal relationships with peers at school, at work, and with friends and partners is substantially reduced if the parent–child relationship is inadequate. Social capital is another important factor to consider (Wilkinson, 1996). The term refers to issues relating to structures where there is a sense of shared norms and values. This creates situations where coordination and cooperation exist for the benefit of society and the creation of civil engagement and better health outcomes. Successful interpersonal skills are required in order for good citizenship to take place. This in turn assists individuals with the potential to offer strong support to others. In the UK in recent years we have seen an alarming increase in the number of crimes and anti-social behaviour amongst our adolescent and teenage populations (Home Office Statistical Bulletin, 2006). Changes in parenting may have contributed to this leading to a focus on parenting and the consequences of poor parenting.

Sub-optimal parenting is more apparent among families living in social deprivation. However, it must be noted that the variation within different social groups is greater than the variation between these groups (Hart and Risley, 1995). Importantly, children experiencing good parenting at home, despite their social and economic environment, are often shielded from the adverse effects that poverty and social deprivation can bring. Conversely, irretrievable damage can be done amongst families where there exist poor inter-parental relationships as well as poor parent–child relationships. It is important to remember the consequences of parental conflict within the family including domestic violence as well as divorcing or separating families (Harold *et al.*, 2001).

Key government documents such as *Choosing Health: Making Healthy Choices Easier* (DH, 2004a) and *Every Child Matters* (DH/DFES, 2004a) identify sub-optimal parenting as one of the determinants of poor physical and mental ill health. Positive parenting is identified as a crucial determinant of emotional and social well-being. Government policy and parenting has also been influenced by some high profile cases such as the deaths of Jamie Bulger (the story is outlined in Chapter 1) and the Victoria Climbié case (Laming, 2003). The Laming Inquiry (2003) recognised the need to address issues relating to vulnerable children and families. Safeguarding and promoting the welfare of children is everybody's business as highlighted in the Children Act (DH, 1989, 2004) and the document *Working Together to Safeguard Children* (HM Govt, 2006). This is all discussed in further depth in Chapters 2 and 9. The implementation of *Every Child Matters* (DH/DfES, 2004a) identified a commitment by the Government to address and support the needs of every child in the country. The Children's agenda arising from this has recognised the need to promote parenting on a universal basis.

The NHS and relevant health care professionals have played a key role in helping these outcomes to be achieved. In conjunction with *Every Child Matters* (DH/DfES, 2004a), the Government has emphasised that the *National Service Framework for Children, Young People and Maternity Services* (NSF) (DH/DfES, 2004b) will feed into the new integrated inspection framework (DfES, 2004b). Additionally, the NSF is closely aligned to the broader *Every Child Matters: Change for Children* (DH/DfES 2004a) implementation programme. Recently, we have seen the integration and implementation of Children's Trusts (DH, 2003) and Children's Centres (DH, 2007a) which have played a key part in the planning, commissioning and delivery of social health, social care and education services. Sure Start has been in existence since 1999 (DfEE, 1999) and supports families living in disadvantaged areas. Information-sharing arrangements between organisations and agencies are improving with the Common Assessment Framework (CAF) (DfES, 2006). Whilst use of this assessment framework is still developing, there is evidence to show that when used appropriately it can have positive holistic benefits for the families concerned. Parenting and parenting capacity are features of the CAF and form a key part of the assessment tool in recognition of the importance of parenting in the health and well-being of children and young people.

The CAF is currently not universally completed and there is much debate as to whether this assessment process should be utilised with all families regardless of their vulnerability. Children's Centres (DH, 2007a), whilst initially being set up in the most deprived and disadvantaged areas, are offering integrated early years education, family and parenting support, as well as the promotion of the facilitation of healthy lifestyles.

The five standards identified in Part 1 of the *National Service Framework for Children, Young People and Maternity Services* (DH/DfES 2004b) have an impact on parenting, directly and indirectly. Standard 1 is particularly relevant to the future health and well-being of children and young people. A key component of this directive facilitates the way forward for the next generation of parents. The new Child Health Promotion Programme (DH/DFES 2004b) puts in place a framework to promote the health and well-being of children and the reduction of health inequalities. It addresses the needs of children from pre-conception through to adulthood, and integrates pre-school and school aged health promotion. Multi-agency health promotion is at the forefront of this programme, ensuring that a range of health and social care practitioners are working together. Children and young people are encouraged to be active in the health care choices they make. They are required to take responsibility for their actions and encouraged to make informed choices about healthy lifestyles. However, universal and targeted health promotion strategies will need to be in place to address the broader determinants of health. This includes providing support for children, including those who are homeless, living in temporary accommodation, and those who have fragile social networks. Access to targeted services will also need to be improved for those where the take-up of services has been poor, such as those not registered with a General Practitioner and for vulnerable families – for example, looked after children, children out of the school setting and children with complex health and social needs. Assessment and early intervention is pivotal to the success of these programmes. The economic studies which have been carried out show that the costs of early intervention with parents are outweighed by future savings in societal costs (Scott *et al.*, 2001b). The earlier the intervention, the better for the parent and child (Marshall and Watt, 1999).

Standard 2 in Part 1 of the NSF (DH/ DFES, 2004b) highlights the importance of positive parenting. It supports the implementation of universal, targeted and specialist services to ensure that parents, including mothers and fathers, receive the required support. This is supported in the Children's Plan (DCSF, 2007) which identifies the need to offer support from infancy through to adulthood to ensure that optimal parenting can take place. There should be support for parents of pre-school children to enable children to make and develop secure emotional and social attachments. This maximises their physical and psychological potential. Support for parents of school-age children should take the form of promoting active parental involvement. The Children's Plan advocated for contracts to be made with parents and better communication once children are in school with the use of 'hand held' records similar to the red book used in the early years. Parents should be encouraged and supported to facilitate the cognitive development of their children, through the stimulation of play and education, as well as dealing with behavioural issues in a positive way. A multi-disciplinary approach should be adopted to direct parents to the appropriate support.

Targeting vulnerable families/communities

In an ideal world, good health should be available for all. Unfortunately, health is not distributed equally and inequalities remain a challenge. A universal approach to the delivery of health care systems is the ideal. However, a small but significant number of families continue to suffer from a large number of problems and are deeply disadvantaged (Cabinet Office, 2006). Mortality rates between routine and manual groups and the population as a whole continue to widen. Between 1997 and 1999 the rate was 13%; however, in 2002–2004 the rate had risen to 19% (DH, 2007c).

There are also parents with specific needs, such as relationship conflict, mental health problems, addiction to drugs or alcohol, teenage parents or parents of disabled children, who should have their needs identified early and be offered intensive multi-agency support. This can be difficult to achieve in hard to reach areas where parents do not access professionals easily. Supporting children and families with complex needs is dicussed further in Chapter 10.

The important issue of the identification of need and the commissioning of appropriate services is addressed in Standards 3 and 5, Part 1 of the NSF (DH/DfES, 2004b). School nurses and health visitors will not be able to fulfil their roles effectively unless this very important issue is addressed. The identification of need, including safeguarding and promoting the welfare of all children, is recognised as a top priority for all agencies. The Government, through the Children's Bill (2004), which became the Children Act (DH, 2004b), requires each local authority to have a Children and Young People's Plan (DfES, 2004). This sets out how the key agencies will work together to safeguard and promote children's welfare. An up-to-date profile of the local population will need to be compiled to facilitate the identification and assessment of children and young people who may be vulnerable and will require input from the agencies concerned. In addition, a community profile is vital for school nurses to profile their schools, and for health visitors to profile their caseloads. Effective supervision should be provided for all agencies who work with children to ensure high quality services are maintained. The Children's Workforce Development Council (CWDC) now has responsibility to develop the knowledge and skills of all professionals working with children and young people. Effective communication and developing partnerships are key skills identified and these can only be achieved by assessing need and targeting services appropriately.

Parenting is at the heart of a number of public health issues, which include eating patterns, obesity, exercise, mental health and delinquency (DH, 2007b). The prevalence of obesity in children under 11 has increased from 9.9% in 1995 to 13.7% in 2003 (Jotangra *et al.*, 2006). Additionally, the rate of psycho-social disorders amongst children is 10–15% in the UK with levels being particularly high in areas of deprivation (DH, 2007c). The issue of supporting and enabling parents to overcome some of these public health concerns through parenting strategies needs to be addressed.

Health visitors and school nurses have always recognised that parents have the greatest impact on a child's life. Warm and positive parenting sets the foundation for optimum health and well-being for life, and mediates the effects of poverty and social disadvantage. There is increasing and compelling neurological evidence that demonstrates how imperative attachment theory is in relation to an infant's neurological development. The components of the brain which control emotional and social development are affected by parent–child relationships very early in life, the first three years being highly significant. Neural pathways established early in life can be changed, but change is more difficult to achieve with increasing age (Shonkoff and Phillips, 2000). This emerging knowledge is likely to have a profound influence on the future role of health visitors and midwives and make early preventative intervention an imperative. Early intervention lays the foundation for future work with parents and families of children and young people of school age.

Engaging parents

The process of engagement is crucial to any form of partnership working successfully. The concept of clients being passive recipients of care no longer exists. It is imperative that the recipients of services are encouraged to participate and negotiate in decision-making processes regarding their own care (McCabe, 2004). So how can parents be engaged?

Firstly, it needs to be acknowledged that there is a changing society with diverse cultural and social needs. In terms of the delivery of care, it needs to be ensured that the services provided put patients, users and the public first. Service provision and service integration needs to be comprehensive and stream lined. It also needs to be accessible, convenient and flexible, enabling more choice for individuals. If the issue of parenting and the engagement of parents is considered, it is vital that this is done in a non-stigmatising way. The availability of services should cover home visiting, as well as those integrated within the communities themselves such as Sure Start and Children's Centres. The Child Health Promotion Programme (CHPP) (DH/DfES, 2004b) is the core health service for protecting, promoting and improving the health and well-being of children. It forms the main health contribution to integrated children's services and its universality is essential. All families will have access to the CHPP, in pregnancy and the first years of life. Successful engagement will further occur if the roles and responsibilities of the service providers are clearly set out, as well as those of the 'user'. It is pivotal that parents realise that the care and support offered to them is unique to their needs.

The Specialist Community Public Health Nursing Courses need to equip health visitors and school nurses to deal with those groups of individuals and families who are difficult to engage (Cabinet Office, 2006). *Facing the Future; a Review of the Role of the Health Visitor* (DH, 2007b, p. 6) described as a priority the need to support the capacity for better parenting:

> ... i.e. improving pregnancy outcomes, child health and development, parents' economic self-sufficiency, safeguarding children, addressing domestic violence, supporting parental relationships and fathers in their parenting role

This can be extended on to the school-age population through liaison with school nurses and education. The Positive Parenting approach to parenting can be facilitated through one-to-one home visiting or through groups. A health care professional works with a parent or family to enable them to address the parenting issues that are giving them concern. Specific parenting programmes will be discussed later in the chapter.

With Positive Parenting many educational group sessions are run jointly by both a health care professional and a parent who has successfully been through a parenting programme. This aspect of engagement is extremely encouraging and it shows other parents how important their contribution is to the development and provision of future services. It is recognised that the needs of fathers have not always been met; they will play a pivotal role in ensuring that the concept of positive parenting applies to both sets of parents. Service provision will therefore need to be more flexible to accommodate the needs of working mothers and fathers. There needs to be a considerable shift away from the concept of 9 a.m. to 5 p.m. working to enable service availability.

Empowering future parents

Among the parents of the future are those currently of school age, and under-standing their needs now and engaging them in order to enable them to be good parents requires a partnership approach. Education and health can work together effectively to ensure that information and support are in place to allow young people to make choices that are right for their age and circum-stances. School nurses are perfectly placed to provide non-judgemental sup-port and information in schools about parenting (DfES/DH, 2006). Building self-esteem and self-confidence are important elements to empowering future parents, which helps to form good child/parent relationships, allowing clear boundaries to be set.

Pregnant teenagers can be supported in the decisions they make through school-based health services, including Extended School services. Health visi-tors, midwives and school nurses can work in partnership to assess and engage teenagers and their families during the antenatal and postnatal period. Health visitors and midwives can then support young people through the transition of pregnancy through to the first years of life. Supporting new parents will also continue in Sure Start areas as well as in the newly formed Children's Centres. Children's Centres are one-stop shops for parents and children, offering early education and child care, family support, health services, employment advice and specialist support on a single site, providing easy access for parents and easy referrals between services (DH, 2007b).

Several parenting programmes exist in order to empower parents of all ages, such as Webster-Stratton and Triple P, which have shown to improve both the short and long term outcomes for children and families (Edwards, *et al.*, 2007). The Nurse Family Partnership Programme in the USA has been a model of care which has worked successfully for vulnerable families over 20 years (Olds *et al.*, 2004). This intensive home visiting programme had 50% better outcomes when nurses delivered the programme. This programme in 2007 was being tested in ten sites across England, with health visitors playing a crucial role in delivering the programme, the results are awaited.

Significant work on positive parenting is being delivered through Extended Schools and After School Clubs, including Youth and Community Centres. Community programmes are more likely to attract parents if provided in the context of other forms of parent support, such as befriending programmes, mutual support groups and drop-in-centres. Such interventions are valued by parents, and improve their mental health and family life. As part of the educa-tional process, it has been recognised that health care professionals are faced with ever-changing public expectations, particularly with regard to choice of health professional and access to different information sources. In addition to programmes and information acquired through television and radio, other information media need to be considered. With the advancement in technology, parents can be engaged using web-based advice and support networks, with assistance given for monitoring their parenting skills and children's development. A considerable number of telephone help lines exist; and could be enhanced through the investment in more resources and staff training. The Government has established the National Families and Parenting Institute (NFPI) and supports a wide range of local and national parenting initiatives through the Parenting Fund, including resource materials and a national helpline for parents. This may be crucial for reaching those parents who will not access other forms of support and enforces the view that a multi-system approach is more effective.

Managing behaviour

Becoming a parent is often described as a joyous and momentous occasion however, the reality for some is very different. There are many factors which can make parenting difficult:

- Negative personal experiences of being parented
- Environmental issues: poverty, social deprivation, poor housing
- Isolation; poor family networks or support
- Poor mental health, including post-natal depression
- Drug and alcohol misuse
- Domestic violence, divorce, separation and lone parenthood
- Having a child with a disability or a complex health need
- Being a young parent or a young person in care
- Having a special educational need or learning disability
- Having a child with a behavioural problem, for example autism
- Having a child with a learning disability

Until there is a clear understanding of some of these difficulties within each individual case, the task of positive parenting will be difficult to achieve (Marshall and Watt, 1999; Gerhardt, 2004). The issue of the behaviour of children and young people creates some difficulties around definitions and there is often conflict between what parents view as poor behaviour and how society views it. Parents may be unaware that their child's behaviour is causing concern until they are placed in a social situation, such as nursery, playgroup or school. Where a child's behaviour is impacting on others would seem to be a good starting point for concern. Alternatively, a parent may have been expressing concerns for some time about their child's behaviour and this should be

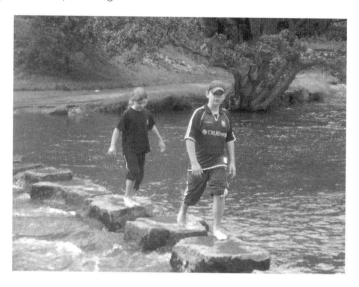

Parenting involves facilitating positive activities

respected and addressed. If it is causing concern for whatever reason, practitioners should take this seriously.

If parents can be facilitated to be confident, with high self-esteem and a clear sense of purpose and direction, there should be similar outcomes for their children. In any behaviour management situation, the crucial aspect is to remain firm and consistent in both actions and statements. Any deviation from this approach will give mixed messages to the child, leading to a sense of frustration for both parties. Therefore, if 'no' is said then it has to mean 'no'. If applying the firm and consistent approach or dealing with any behavioural issue, it is critical that all those involved in parenting deal with the same situation in the same way. Children thrive when they have clear boundaries and expectations that they can work towards, but it needs to be highlighted that any boundaries set should be age-appropriate for that child. It is helpful for parents to have knowledge of the developmental stages that children go through, to enable them to set age-appropriate goals and behavioural boundaries.

When children are clear about what is expected of them in given situations, whether at home, in social settings or at school, then their ability to conform is easier, and the child will feel more confident in carrying out the adult's wishes. Difficulties arise when boundaries are continuously changed; the child's confidence is quickly eroded and the child is less likely to conform to the wishes of the adult. The child's behaviour then becomes more challenging and often spirals out of control. The issue of respect also loses its significance and this is a two-way process. It is important that the issue of respect is maintained for both the parent and child, which is fundamental to the parent–child relationship. This is particularly true as the child grows up. Adolescent behaviour will often push the boundaries set by parents and dealing with this in a respect-ful way using effective communication is vital to success. In school, it is a common problem expressed by teenagers that adults do not show them respect and make assumptions about their behaviour, which is both frustrating and likely to compound poor behaviour.

The concept of positive parenting relies on parents having the ability to remain confident in their actions even when things go wrong. Key to this idea is positive reinforcement. Parents can place a huge value on their children by rewarding good behaviour and ignoring bad behaviour. More often than not it is the bad behaviour that is rewarded, in the sense that attention is drawn to this. If a child is lacking in any form of attention but gets a response through bad behaviour, the child will see this as some kind of reward. The situation can then become a self-fulfilling prophecy as the child will continue to behave badly. Giving children age-appropriate responsibilities and praising them for their efforts is a positive way of building up their self-esteem and confidence. For older children and adolescents, this is particularly important as they become independent from their parents and need to be trusted to achieve on their own.

Positive reinforcement can occur in very simple ways, such as giving praise, paying them a compliment, and even rewarding them for accepting what you say, being reasonable and behaving well. Getting the balance right between love and discipline is not an easy task; the majority of parents struggle to get this right and some need to resort to health care professionals for advice. Par-ents need to be assured that they are not bad parents and that as children grow up the tensions in the family can grow and cause conflict. Reassurance that setting firm boundaries, listening to children and young people and respecting them as individuals is key.

When positive parenting breaks down or situations occur where the child refuses to cooperate, it is advisable to stay in control. Some parents utilise 'time out' strategies, where either the child is removed from the situation or the parent removes themselves. Older children may have their privileges removed over a certain time frame. It is important that the child is informed that their behaviour is unacceptable. The consequences of that behaviour continuing also need to be explained and the child has the option to stop or continue. Children need to realise that, as a consequence of choosing to continue with their bad behaviour, privileges can be denied.

In terms of behaviour management, two complementary theoretical sys-tems are generally followed. They take the form of a behavioural and a rela-tionship approach (Stewart-Brown, 2005). The behavioural approach aims to help parents develop positive discipline strategies by building a good relation-ship with their child through, for example, child-led play, setting clear bounda-ries and enforcing them without physical or emotional violence. The relation-ship approach aims to build parents' emotional awareness of their children and themselves, increasing respect and empathy for children, and developing their capacity to nurture themselves as well as their children (Wolfendale and Einzig, 1999). Many parenting programmes follow the above theoretical components and almost all programmes teach positive discipline.

Parenting programmes can be effective in groups, where parents can share experiences and try different techniques that other parents have tried. However, for some parents, groups are too intimidating and they are more comfortable on a one-to-one basis. For example, teenage parents may be uncomfortable in a group with older mums. Whatever the situation, the most effective results will be where trust is developed with the parent and this is not always the health professional. People from a range of backgrounds, health visiting, school nursing, the voluntary and charitable sector, social work, and clinical psychology have provided successful and long-term interventions in the past. It is the skill of the facilitator that is paramount to the success of parenting programmes or interventions. An approach which aims to empower parents by forming a partnership which builds on the strengths rather than the weaknesses of parents will be most effective. Many parents will not engage in 'parenting skills' training as they feel that they are being judged and so this aspect is very important in the building of trust.

A considerable number of parenting programmes exist. However, the Webster-Stratton Parenting Programme has been useful across the range of behavioural problems including those with specific behavioural difficulties such as Attention Deficit Hyperactivity Disorder (ADHD), autism or other learning disabilities. Enabling parents to learn positive, non-coercive discipline, and to improve the quality of their relationships with their children, are key aims of behavioural parenting programmes. Controlled trials demonstrate these programmes to be effective in reducing behaviour problems (Webster-Stratton *et al.*, 1989; Serketich and Dumas, 1996; Dimond and Hyde, 1999; Barlow and Stewart-Brown, 2000; Scott *et al.*, 2001), as well as improving the mental health of parents (Barlow *et al.*, 2002). Parenting programmes therefore have a potentially important role to play in child health and mental health promotion programmes.

The school nurse and the health visitor will play a pivotal part in the delivery of such parenting programmes. It has been suggested that for maximum effectiveness, these programmes may need to be offered to all parents (Stewart-Brown, 1989; Hall and Elliman, 2003). The Webster-Stratton parenting programme consists of four modules. The parents are given step-by-step guidance and there is a focus on the following elements:

- Playing with children
- Helping them learn
- Using praise and rewards
- Setting limits and handling behaviour

Parents are taught very specific skills and such elements are displayed visually in the form of a pyramid where one technique builds on previous ones. The programme consists of 2 hour sessions, once a week, for a span of 10 weeks. The activities include video vignettes of parent–child interactions, group discussion, role-play, rehearsal of parenting techniques, and home practice. Each parenting group is run by a school nurse or health visitor with another health care professional as co-leader. All group leaders receive three days of training in programme delivery from the Family Nurturing Network (FNN) in Oxford. The FNN is a voluntary organisation working primarily with families referred by social workers or self-referred for child behaviour problems. All the group leaders receive weekly group supervision with a clinical psychologist.

With regard to other parenting programmes, a study by Barlow and Stewart-Brown (2001) found that the Family Links parenting programme benefited parents through improved mutual support, brought a sense of normality to problems, helped parents to regain a sense of control in relation to parenting, increased their ability to cope in a calm way, increased their practical skills, improved the parent–child relationship, and increased their empathy and emotional understanding. Further studies on Parenting Programmes by Grimshaw and McGuire (1998); and Mockford and Barlow (2004) concern the need for partners to attend such programmes and for there to be continued support after completion of the programme. Many parents indicated in these studies that making changes would have been easier if their partners had attended the programme with them.

Conclusion

This chapter has explored the complex issue of parenting in the 21st century. The Government has acknowledged the devastating effects that sub-optimal parenting can have on society as a whole. Key policies have been designed to address, both directly and indirectly, the issue of parenting. What is clear is that positive parenting is everyone's business. Health visitors and school nurses should be proud that they will be involved strategically in delivering future early intervention parenting programmes and school health initiatives, at both community and individual levels. The government recognises that a variety of different workers have a role to play in working with children, young adults and parents to enable them to attain optimal parenting skills. It is also an opportunity to lessen the gap in terms of health inequalities and to help those disadvantaged families. Despite the fact that the resource implications of the recommended Government initiatives are high, it is hoped that the benefits of such parenting programme initiatives and government schemes will eventually outweigh the costs to society on a grand scale. This is an exciting and challenging time for all health and social care practitioners. It will involve collaborative working in its widest sense, with parents, children and young adults playing a key role. It is time to embrace change and to work in partnership with the parents and children of today and the future.

References

Barlow, J. and Stewart-Brown, S. (2000) Behaviour problems and parent education programmes. *Developmental and Behavioural Paediatrics*, **21**, 356–70.

Barlow, J. and Stewart-Brown, S. (2001) Understanding parenting programmes: parents' views. *Primary Health Care Research and Development*, **2**, 117–30.

Barlow, J., Coren, E. and Stewart-Brown, S. (2002) Meta-analysis of the effectiveness of parenting programmes in improving maternal psychosocial health. *British Journal of General Practice*, **52**, 223–33.

Cabinet Office (2006) *Reaching Out: Social Exclusion Action Plan*. Stationery Office, London.

Children's Bill (2004) The UK parliament. http://www.publications.parliament.co.uk/; accessed 30 December 2007.

Children's Workforce Development Council (CWDC) http://www.cwdcouncil.org.uk/.

Collins Pocket English Dictionary (2000) HarperCollins, London.

Department for Children, Schools and Families (2007) *The Children's Plan: Building Brighter Futures*. DCSF, London.

Department for Education and Employment (DfEE 1999*) Sure Start: Making A Difference for Children and Families*. DfEE, London.

Department for Education and Skills (2004) *Children and Young People's Plan*. DfES, London.

Department for Education and Skills (2004b) *Every Child Matters: Change for Children in Schools: a Summary of DFES Guidance*. DFES, London.

Department for Education and Skills (2006) *Evaluating the Common Assessment Framework and Lead Professional Guidance and Implementation in 2005–2006*. http://www.dfespublications.gov.uk/; accessed 30 December 2007.

Department for Education and Skills, Department of Health (2006) *The School Nurse Practice Development Resource Pack*. DfES, DH, London.

Department of Health/Department for Education and Skills (2004a) *Every Child Matters: Change for Children*. DH, London.

Department of Health/Department for Education and Skills (2004b) *National Service Framework for Children, Young People and Maternity Services*. DH, London.

Department of Health (1989) *The Children Act*. DH, London.

Department of Health (2003) *Children's Trusts*. DH, London.

Department of Health (2004a) *Choosing Health: Making Healthier Choices Easier*. DH, London.

Department of Health (2004b) *The Children Act*. DH, London.

Department of Health (2007a) *Delivering Health Services Through Sure Start Children's Centres*. DH, London.

Department of Health (2007b) *Facing the Future: a Review of the Role of Health Visitors*. DH, London.

Department of Health (2007c) *Review of the Health Inequalities Infant Mortality PSA Target*. DH, London.

Dimond, C. and Hyde, C. (1999) *Report No.19, interTasc no. 26/1999*. West Midlands Development and Evaluation Service, University of Birmingham.

Edwards, R. T. Ceilleachair, A., Bywater, T., Hughes, D. A. and Hutchings, J. (2007) Parenting programme for parents of children at risk of developing conduct disorder: cost effectiveness analysis. *British Medical Journal*, **334**, 682.

Gerhardt, S. (2004). *Why Love Matters*. Routledge, London.

Giddens, A. (2006) *Sociology*, 5th edn. Polity, Cambridge.

Grimshaw, R. and McGuire, C. (1998) *Evaluating Parenting Programmes: a Study of Stakeholder's Views*. National Children's Bureau, London.

Hall, D. and Elliman, D. (2003) *Health for All Children*, 4th edn. Oxford University Press, Oxford.

Hardyment, C. (1995) *Perfect Parents. Baby Care Past and Present*. Oxford University Press, Oxford.

Harold, G., Pryor, J. and Reynolds, J. (2001) *Not in Front of the Children? How Conflict Between Parents Affects Children*. One Plus One, London.

Hart, B. and Risley, T. R. (1995) *Meaningful Differences in the Everyday Experience of Young American Children*. Paul H. Brookes, Baltimore.

HM Government (2006) *Working Together to Safeguard Children: A Guide to Interagency Working to Safeguard and Promote the Welfare of Children*. HM Government, London.

Home Office Statistical Bulletin (2006) *Young People and Crime, Findings from the 2005 Offending, Crime and Justice Survey*. Home Office, London.

Jotangra, D., Moody, A., Stamatakis, E. and Wardle, H. (2006) *Obesity Among Children Under 11*. DH, London.

Laming, H. (2003) *The Victoria Climbié Inquiry, Report of an Inquiry*. Department of Health and Home Office, London.

Olds, D. L., Robinson, J., Pettitt, L., Luckey, D. W., Holmberg, J., Ng, K., Isacks, R., Sheff, K. and Henderson, C. R. (2004) Effects of home visits by paraprofessionals and by nurses: age 4 follow-up results of a randomized trial. *Pediatrics*, **114**(6), 1560–8.

Marshall, J. and Watt, P. (1999) *Child Behaviour Problems: A Literature Review of the Size and Nature of the Problem and Prevention Interventions in Childhood*. The Inter Agency Committee on Children's Futures, Perth.

McCabe, C. (2004) Nurse–patient communication: an exploration of patients' experiences. *Journal of Clinical Nursing*, **13**, 41–9.

Mockford, C. and Barlow, J. (2004) Parenting programmes: some unintended consequences. *Primary Care Research and Development*, **5**, 219–27.

Royal College of Paediatrics and Child Health (2002) *Helpful Parenting*. Royal College of Paediatrics and Child Health, London.

Sanders, M. R. and Christensen, A. P. (1985) A comparison of the effects of child management and planned activities training in five parenting environments. *Journal of Abnormal Child Psychology*, **13**, 101–17.

Scott, S., Spender, Q., Doolan, M., Jacobs, B. and Aspland, H. (2001a) Multicentre controlled trial of parenting groups for childhood antisocial behaviour in clinical practice. *British Medical Journal*, **32**, 194–8.

Scott, S., Knapp, M., Henderson, J. and Maughan, B. (2001b) Financial cost of social exclusion: follow up study of antisocial children into adulthood. *British Medical Journal*, **323**, 1–5.

Serkeitch, W. and Dumas, J. (1996) The effectiveness of behavioural parent training to modify anti-social behaviour in children: a meta-analysis. *Behaviour Therapy*, **27**, 171–86.

Shaw, R. and Stewart-Brown, S. L. (2004) The roots of social capital: relationships in the home during childhood and health in later life. In *Social Capital for Health: Issues of Definition, Measurement and Links to Health* (eds. A. Morgan and C. Swann). Health Development Agency, London.

Shonkoff, J. and Phillips, D. (2000) *From Neurons to Neighbourhoods: the Science of Early Childhood Development*. National Academy Press, Washington DC.

Shore, R. (1997) *Rethinking the Brain: New Insights Into Early Development*. New York Families and Work Institute, New York.

Stewart-Brown, S. (1989) Public health implications of childhood behaviour problems and parenting programmes. In: *Parenting, Schooling and Children's Behaviour* (eds. A. Buchanan and B. Hudson). Ashgate Publishing, Aldershot.

Stewart-Brown, S. (2000) Parenting, well-being, health and disease In: *Promoting Children's Emotional Well-Being* (eds. A. Buchanan and B. Hudson). Oxford University Press, Oxford.

Stewart-Brown, S. (2005) Mental health promotion – childhood holds the key. *Public Health Medicine*, **5**(3), 8–17.

Webster-Stratton, C., Holingsworth, T. and Kolpacoff, M. (1989) The long term effectiveness and clinical significance of three cost effective training programmes for families with conduct-problem children. *Journal of Consult Clinical Psychology*, **57**, 550–3.

Wilkinson, R. (1996) *Unhealthy Societies*. Routledge, London.

Wisensale, S. K. (1992) Toward the 21st century: family change and public policy. *Family Relations*, **41**(4), 417–22.

Wolfendale, S. and Einzig, H. (1999) *Parenting Education and Support: New Opportunities*. David Fulton, London.

Useful websites

The Incredible Years: Reducing children's aggression and increasing social competence at home and school (Webster-Stratton): http://www.incredibleyears.com/

Sure Start: http://www.surestart.gov.uk/

Triple P: Positive Parenting Programme: http://www.triplep.net/

CHAPTER 7

Mental health and well-being of children and young people

Gill Coverdale

Key themes

- Definition of mental health and mental ill health
- Incidence and impact of mental ill health
- Practical advice on enhancing mental health and emotional well-being and building resilience
- Guidance on managing mental ill health and the support services available

> The true measure of a nation's standing is how well it attends to its children – their health and safety, their material security, their education and socialization, and their sense of being loved, valued, and included in the families and societies into which they are born (United Nations Children's Fund [UNICEF], 2007).

Introduction

The Every Child Matters [ECM] agenda aims to ensure that children and young people grow up feeling safe, valued and comfortable with themselves as a person and are more able to achieve, contribute, make healthy choices and enjoy life in the process (Department of Health [DH], Department of Education and Skills [DfES], 2003). With ECM targets to be met by 2010, and in order to achieve the above potential, those people working with children and young people require an understanding of what being mentally healthy is and a knowledge of the difference between problems and disorders.

What is mental health?

Mental health is about being physically and emotionally healthy, having the strength and the capacity to live a full and creative life, and the flexibility to deal with its ups and downs (Young Minds, 2006). It is normal for the average teenager to worry about their looks, relationships with family and friends, school, and career, as a modicum of worry and anxiety helps prepare them for life events. UNICEF (2007) has recently published its report on the findings of a comprehensive assessment into the health and well-being of children, young people and their families in the 21 most developed countries. The United Kingdom [UK] and the United States [US] were in the bottom third of the rankings for five of the six dimensions reviewed in the assessment. This is a sad indictment of a developed and resource-rich society.

The relationships that children develop with their family and friends are very important in both their present and future lives and have an impact on emotional health and well-being. UNICEF (2007) measured the strength of family structure, relationships with parents and relationships with friends and peers, to arrive at a combined overview of the 'relationships' dimension of child well-being. The UK is bottom of the chart in this and the behaviours and risks section. This is a vital aspect of children's and young people's childhood experience; the World Health Organization states that 'Being liked and accepted by peers' is 'crucial to young people's health and development, and those who are not socially integrated are far more likely to exhibit difficulties with their physical and emotional health' (UNICEF, 2007, p. 25).

What is mental ill health?

Mental health problems are the largest single cause of illness and disability in England (Johnson, 2007). Mental health problems in children and young people may be defined as abnormalities of emotions, behaviour or social relationships, which become sufficiently marked or prolonged, resulting in suffering or risk to optimal development in the child, or distress or disturbance in the family or community (Young Minds, 2006). Table 7.1 shows the types of problems/disorders associated with mental ill health.

Most mental disorders begin between the ages of 12 and 24 years, but are often left undetected until later in life (Patel *et al.*, 2007). It is acknowledged that recognising mental health issues in children and young people and separating mental illness and mental distress is a difficult task (DeBell and Tomkins, 2006). Careful assessment and management, or appropriate referral,

Table 7.1 Common mental health problems.

■ Behaviour problems	■ Self-harm/suicidal behaviour
■ Sleep problems	■ Depression
■ Phobias	■ Asperger's/autism
■ Social anxieties	■ Learning disabilities (LD)
■ Abdominal pains	■ Eating disorders (bulimia, anorexia)
■ Bedwetting/soiling	
■ Obsessive Compulsive Disorder (OCD)	■ Conduct disorders such as: defiance; anti-social and aggressive behaviour
■ Attention Deficit Hyperactive Disorder (ADHD)	■ Enuresis and encoperesis

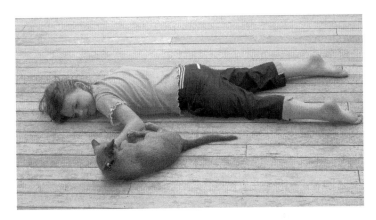

Positive relationships encourage well being

require the skills and knowledge of those 'professionals' involved. CAMHS do not regard behaviour and sleep problems, phobias and social anxieties as a priority; rather, self-harm, depressive behaviour, Attention Deficit Hyperactive Disorder [ADHD], autism, Learning Disability [LD] and eating disorders are disorders that need to be referred.

Society's perception of mental health

Health professionals, educationalists, social workers and psychologists use various terminology to describe mental health problems, referring to risk, developmental harm and challenging behaviour (Young Minds, 2007), so it is most important that professionals explore shared terminology and assumptions. Very often the word 'mental' has a negative connotation which results in people having a degree of ignorance about what being mentally healthy is and a degree of intolerance, or fear, of mental ill health. This can result in inadequate attention being paid to any problems arising, resulting in them escalating to crisis point before they are addressed.

Despite advances in the layperson's perspectives about their health, mental health still has a stigma (Patel *et al.*, 2007). The government campaign 'Mind out for Mental Health', launched in 2001 with the *Journey to Recovery* policy document (DH, 2001), challenged the discrimination caused by mental ill health, calling for awareness raising and promotion of mental health and well-being to be carried out in a range of settings, including schools, workplaces, prisons and the media. In addition to this it aims to raise awareness of common mental ill health disorders and to provide early signposting to advice services to prevent escalating mental ill health in children and young people.

In 2001, the Department of Health argued that psychoses often begin developing in the teenage years, but it took six to twelve months for help to be received (DH, 2001). They called for support for those agencies coming into first contact with teenagers. Recent research has shown that most mental health needs in young people remain unmet largely due to a shortage of mental health professionals, low capacity of non-specialist mental health professionals and the poor quality of mental health services for children and young people (Patel *et al.*, 2007). The Department of Health has recently commissioned the development of a dataset for use in England to support the implementation of Standard 9 of the National Service Framework [NSF] for Children, Young People and Maternity Services (DH/DfES, 2004c). This is the latest set of standards on the delivery of a comprehensive CAMHS.

The incidence of mental ill health

Table 7.2 shows the range of prevalence statistics gathered by the varying forums, charities and organisations who support and carry out research into child and adolescent mental health.

Risky behaviours and risk factors

There is a strong correlation between the prevalence of social problems, risky behaviour and reduced child well-being and much has been written and researched (Wanless, 2004; DH/DfES, 2004c; Patel *et al.*, 2007; Young Minds,

Table 7.2 Facts and figures.

Facts and figures from Young Minds (2007)

- 20–30% of children aged between 4 and 20 years have a mental health problem
- 10% of 5–15 year olds in the UK have some type of mental disorder
- 5% have a clinically significant conduct disorder
- 4% are assessed as having emotional disorders (anxiety and depression)
- 1% are rated as hyperkinetic (disturbances of activity or attention)

Facts and figures from the Child Mental Health Centre (2007)

- British young people are involved in more violence, drug taking and binge drinking than teenagers in other European countries
- 168,000 11–15 year olds abused glue and solvents in the last year
- The average onset age of self-harm is 12
- 1 in 5 girls (aged 15–17) self-harm
- Suicide rates start to increase from age 11
- On average, a teenager tries to kill themselves every 22 minutes
- A third of all boys and a quarter of all girls will bully other children at some time in their school career
- Over 40,000 children are prescribed anti-depressants in the UK
- There are over 30,000 children and young people on waiting lists for mental health services in the UK
- Nearly half of all teenagers say they are unable to talk to their parents about their problems
- In a quarter of the country, there is no emergency help for severely depressed teenagers and many GPs are being forced to prescribe anti-depressants to children and young people, against NICE guidelines, as waiting lists for psychological therapies are so long

2007). It is also acknowledged that social problems often reflect circumstances, pressures, and self-perceptions that undermine well-being (Young Minds, 2007). UNICEF (2007) suggests that risky behaviour indicates problems and pressures facing a significant proportion of young people and the inability to cope with such pressures. The UK finds itself at the foot of the risky behaviours tables (UNICEF, 2007) and Table 7.3 provides information on the high-risk behaviours of UK young people captured by the report.

Mental health problems are also acknowledged to increase the incidence of other risky behaviours, such as eating disorders and obesity, deviant behaviour, school phobia/social phobia and crime. It is accepted that these behaviours can also cause mental health problems.

Townley (2002) describes the following risk factors associated with poor mental health:

- genetic influences
- low self-esteem
- overt parental conflict
- socio-economic disadvantage
- having a learning disability
- abusive relationships (such as domestic violence in the home; child abuse – physical, sexual or emotional)

UNICEF (2007, p. 32) suggests that children who witness violence in the home are also most likely to be victims of violence themselves, leading to 'incalculable levels of current misery and long-term damage' to the emotional well-being of many children. Bullying is experienced by between a third and a half of all pupils as either victims or perpetrators (DH/DfES, 2004b). It is also a major contributor to poor self-image, esteem and belief in one's self as a valuable person. It can have a major impact on a person for the rest of their life, affecting emotional health and problems such as anxiety and depression. Children view addressing the problem of bullying along with violence and abuse as a top priority for their emotional well-being (DH, 2007). Tackling bullying during childhood is imperative and the National Healthy Schools Programme

Table 7.3 High-risk behaviours (Child Mental Health Centre, 2007).

- 30% of young people report being drunk on two or more occasions
- 30% of 15 year-olds have used cannabis (regular cannabis use is associated with depression and problems at school, and could trigger psychoses in young people prone to such conditions)
- 40% of young people have had sexual intercourse by the age of 15
- Young people who smoke cigarettes, for example, are approximately three times more likely to use alcohol regularly and eight times more likely to use cannabis.

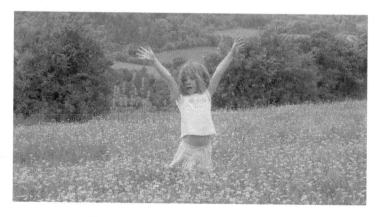

Physical activity raises self-esteem.

(DH/DfES, 2004a) has specifically addressed bullying in its *Promoting Emotional Health and Well-Being* document (DH/DfES, 2004b).

Children's and young people's emotional well-being is closely linked to their subjective view of their psychological and social well-being. Feelings of awkwardness, loneliness, and 'being an outsider' – their perceptions of social exclusion – can significantly affect the quality of young people's lives (UNICEF, 2007). The UNICEF (2007) report's main aim was to identify whether children feel loved, cherished, special and supported, within the family and community, and whether the family and community are being supported in this task by public policy and resources. The UK came bottom of all the countries in this category.

Social inequalities in mental health

Poverty, as seen by Acheson (1998) and Wanless (2004), as well as affecting physical health and development, can have lasting damage on cognitive development, achievement at school, aspirations, self-perceptions, relationships, risk behaviours and employment prospects. Children in social class V are three times more likely to have a mental health problem than those in social class I and there are higher rates of schizophrenia, alcoholism and organic psychosis in poorer areas (Young Minds, 2007). Being born on the wrong side of the health divide has a lasting and intergenerational impact and the government has committed to improving emotional well-being and tackling poor mental health in deprived communities as central to reducing health inequalities (Johnson, 2007).

There are gender differences too, with the greatest differential being in schizophrenia and suicide in young men, which is the second most common cause of death among young men (DH, 1999). This is reducing gradually (Young Minds, 2006), but for the black and ethnic minority population the incidence of mental ill health can be nine times higher than the rest of the population. Access to mental health services is unequal, Asian people are less likely to be offered therapy and black people are more likely to be compelled to take treatments (Johnson, 2007). The government is committed to addressing this through its new policy on improving mental health services for black and minority ethnic communities (National Institute for Mental Health in England [NIMHE], 2007).

The policy influence

Mental health is one of the government's key priorities as outlined in the NHS Plan (DH, 2000). There is a plethora of policy addressing both the promotion of

Table 7.4 The policy influence.

- DH (1999) *National Service Framework for Mental Health*
- DH & DfEE (1999) *The National Healthy Schools Standard*
- DH (1999a) *Saving Lives – Our Healthier Nation*
- DH (1999b) *Making a Difference: Strengthening the Nursing, Midwifery and Health Visiting Contributions to Health and Healthcare*
- DH (2001) *Health Visitor Practice Development Resource Pack*
- DfES (2003) *Every Child Matters*
- DH & CPHVA (2003) *Liberating the Public Health Talents of Community Practitioners and Health Visitors*
- DH (2004a) *Choosing Health. Making Healthier Choices Easier*
- DH (2004b) *The Chief Nursing Officer's Review of the Nursing, Midwifery and Health Visiting Contribution to Vulnerable Children and Young People*
- DfES (2004) *Healthy Living Blueprint*
- DH & DfES (2004) *Every Child Matters – The Next Steps*
- DH & DfES (2004) *National Service Framework for Children and Maternity Services*
- DH & DfEE (2004) *Promoting Emotional Health and Well-Being Through the National Healthy School Standard*
- DH, DfES (2004) *National Healthy Schools Programme*
- NICE (2005) *Depression in Children and Young People*
- DH (2006) *School Nurse Practice Development Resource Pack*
- National Institute for Mental Health in England (2007) *Inside Outside: Improving Mental Health Services for Black and Minority Ethnic Communities in England*

mental health and reducing the morbidity associated with mental ill health. All the papers listed in Table 7.4 have sections addressing mental health promotion and prevention, advocating the encouragement and facilitation of healthy and active lifestyles, which involves increasing self-esteem, confidence, self-belief and psychological well-being. Good self-belief and self-esteem are major contributors to healthy mental well-being.

Prevention and promotion

Mental health commissioning is still dominated by services to treat mental illness. It is rare that commissioners work together to build services to promote mental well-being or to address the wider needs of people with either severe or common mental health problems. (Sainsbury Centre for Mental Health [SCMH], 2007)

Many people, including parents, relatives, siblings, teachers, learning mentors and organisations linked to children and young people have a direct interest in the emotional and mental well-being of children and young people. If a child or young person is angry, bewildered, bereaved, stressed or worried in any way, then many people are affected in the fallout of such emotions. It is important that everyone is prepared to promote and support healthy mental and emotional development and be able to address problems before they become crises.

Raising awareness of what being mentally healthy is and reducing the stigma of mental ill health can be addressed by covering topics associated with mental health and emotional well-being in school through the Personal, Social, Health and Citizenship curriculum. Drama, case studies, discussion and debate, circle time and role-play can all help to raise awareness, raise self-esteem and change the perception of mental health being linked to 'madness' and 'badness' (DH/DfES, 2004b).

Emotional well-being is said to be achieved when a child feels happy, calm and confident (DH/DfES, 2004b). Positive experiences such as being praised, solving problems with others, having friends and someone to talk to and being a successful learner are all things that young people feel have a positive impact on their emotional well-being (Ahmad *et al.*, 2003). Positive emotions can ensure that deep transferrable learning occurs, and this in turn promotes a healthy mind and body and a sense of security and happiness (Barnes, 2005). All this in turn will help raise self-esteem and provide a strong sense of self-worth and the strength to manage strong feelings, deal with and resolve conflict and recover from setbacks. Effective promotion of mental and emotional well-being also fosters in young people an understanding of the feelings of others and empathy to show care and concern.

The Health Development Agency (DH, DfES, 2004b) has identified that promoting emotional health and well-being contributes significantly to all the ECM outcomes for children and young people and helps children and young people to understand and express their feelings, build their confidence and emotional resilience, and therefore their capacity to learn. To this end, ten aspects, which include policy and curriculum development as well as assessing the school culture and provision of support services, have been identified to be integral to a whole school approach to promoting emotional health and well-being and addressing bullying (DH, DfES 2004b) and are linked to the achievement of the National Healthy Schools Standard and Office for Standards in Education [Ofsted].

There are numerous resources to aid the promotion of mental health and emotional well-being with children, young people and parents and some of these links can be found in Table 7.5.

Table 7.5 Resource sources for promoting mental health and emotional well-being.

- DH & DfEE (2004) *Promoting Emotional Health and Well-being Through the National Healthy School Standard*
- Wired for Health: http://www.wiredforhealth.gov.uk/
- National Healthy Schools Programme: http://www.healthyschools.gov.uk/
- The Sainsbury Centre for Mental Health: http://www.scmh.org.uk/
- The Association for Child and Adolescent Mental Health (ACAMH): http://www.acamh.org.uk/
- Mental Health Foundation Children and Young People: http://www.mentalhealth.org.uk/information/mental-health-a-z/children-and-young-people
- Royal College of Psychiatrists: www.rcpsych.ac.uk/info/mhgu/newm-hgu14.htm
- Bullying UK: http://www.bullying.co.uk/
- Young Minds: http://www.youngminds.org.uk/

These resources also acknowledge the contribution that parents make to developing their children's mental and emotional well-being, and therefore supporting parental emotional well-being and helping them to manage and enjoy their children is also imperative.

Identification of common mental health problems

It has already been acknowledged that early identification of mental illness is necessary by those having first contact with children and young people in distress. Separating out low mood and slippage into mental ill health is difficult, but Whooley *et al.* (1997) offer the Two Question Test for screening, arguing that these questions are more effective than a barrage of questions:

> During the last month, have you often been bothered by feeling down, depressed or hopeless?

> During the last month, have you often been bothered by little interest or pleasure in doing things?

Parents also need support from professionals if they seek help about their child. If early interventions are put in place and children and young people encouraged to seek help early, it could be argued there would be a good outcome.

This chapter will not address severe and enduring mental illness, but guidance on key issues experienced by those working with children and young people will be addressed, albeit briefly, with signposting to further resources. Readers' attention is drawn to the National Institute for Health and Clinical Excellence [NICE] clinical guidelines on Eating Disorders (NICE, 2004a); Self Harm (NICE, 2004b) and Depression (NICE, 2005). The excellent document *Drawing on the Evidence* (Wolpert *et al.*, 2006) and the *Making it Work Guide* (Frank, 2002) plus the resources section offered in Table 7.5 are invaluable, as is the Young Minds website which offers free and confidential advice for non-specialist professionals, families and young people.

Behavioural problems

Behaviour develops from a very young age and is closely influenced by the interactions that children have with their parents/carers and any traumatic events that happen. It is also affected by the attachments children have in the very early stages in life. There are many behavioural problems affecting children and young people from anxiety and conduct disorders to anti-social behaviour and youth offending. Early identification and help exploring the underlying explanations using a multi-disciplinary approach is the best action (Young Minds, 2007).

Obsessive Compulsive Disorder (OCD)

Geller *et al.* (1998) suggest that 1–4% of children, adolescents and adults exhibit Obsessive Compulsive behaviour – a psychological disorder based on learning processes. There are theorists (Salkovskis *et al.*, 1999) who purport that children and young people may have OCD due to their parents' own over-anxious psychological state and their feelings that the world is a dangerous place. Derisley *et al.*'s (2005) study examined parental incidence of OCD and other anxiety states and found that the adolescents of those parents with anxiety and obsessive disorders did have poorer mental health and called for involvement of families in treatments for OCD in the child and adolescent population. The NICE guidelines on Anxiety Disorders (2004c) offer clear direction for adult sufferers, but none on children or adolescents, who will require referral on to CAMHS.

Self-harm

The NICE guidelines (NICE, 2004b) on Self Harm define it as 'self poisoning or injury, irrespective of the apparent purpose of the act'. It has many antecedent causes such as abuse (sexual, physical and emotional), depression, mood disorders, loss and bereavement and parental mental illness (Mental Health Foundation, 2007c; Favazza, 1996; Preece and Jowett, 2007). It can lead to a sense of hopelessness, poor relationships, difficulties at school and at its most extreme it leads to delusional behaviour, attempted suicide and death (NICE, 2004b; Souter and Kramer, 2004). Souter and Kramer (2004) argue that the incidence of overdosing and suicide in young people is very low at between 4 and 11% and that it is most unlikely that psychotic young people self-harm. It appears that in most cases self-harm is an expression of personal distress (NICE, 2004b), a systematic cry for help. NICE (2004b) have produced guidelines for its management and Souter and Kramer (2004) propose a child protection approach to dealing with children and young people presenting with self-harming behaviour.

The key aspects of managing these distressed youngsters are to listen to them and hear their story, which requires respect and sympathy. A measurement of how suicidal the young person is and an understanding of the precipitating factors, are both necessary in deciding on management, and whether there needs to be admission to hospital or referral on to specialist CAMHS. Addressing the cause and psychotherapeutic counselling can lead to a good outcome. It is clear from the literature that staff training on managing the immediate impact of self-harm is necessary for all those working with children and young people (NICE, 2004b).

Depression

Depression is the persistent exaggeration of the everyday feelings that accompany sadness (Mental Health Foundation, 2007a). It may start with an alteration in mood resulting in low spirits, loss of interest, tearfulness, anxiety and sleep problems to feelings of hopelessness and suicide. Young children tend to exhibit their low mood through physical pain such as stomach aches or headaches, and may not be able to articulate their feelings, whereas older children may be able to talk about how sad they are feeling. Close attention should be paid to these indicators, especially if they are repetitious or prolonged.

NICE (2005) have produced a quick reference guide for the identification and management of children and young people with depression in primary, community and secondary care. This excellent resource takes the reader through the recognition, assessment and treatment options for the different levels of practitioner utilising the tiered CAMHS approach. It advises key priorities for implementation that include recording the child or young person's co-morbidities, social, educational and family context for the patient and the family. Cognitive Behavioural Therapy [CBT] is a popular approach used by

Tier 2 CAMHS; it is a 'talking treatment' attempting to alter the way people feel and think about themselves and helping them to challenge the negative thoughts.

Eating disorders

The most common eating disorders seen in young people are Anorexia Nervosa and Bulimia Nervosa, which occur in 2% of the female adult population (Mental Health Foundation, 2007b). Anorexia is when the sufferer does not eat enough because of the way they feel about themselves or how they look, which is often distorted. It can lead to brittle bones, kidney disease, hormonal disorders and hair loss. Bulimia is when sufferers binge and then feel out of control and make themselves sick or use a large amount of laxatives, which can lead to tooth decay, constipation and intestinal damage (Mental Health Foundation, 2007b).

NICE (2004a) have produced guidance on the treatment and management of eating disorders and Young Minds (2007) suggests that children and young people need access to services where they can be listened to and helped to explore the underlying concerns, with an early referral on to specialist CAMH services for CBT.

Substance misuse

Vimpani (2005) suggests that little attention is paid to the upstream events that lead to substance misuse, as most attention goes into either prohibition or harm minimisation. He argues that substance misuse correlates strongly with adverse life outcomes, such as unemployment and antisocial behaviour. He cites a growing body of evidence pointing to the benefits of risk minimisation and protection enhancement embedded into family and social systems, as the essential building blocks of a set of early intervention strategies that begin in the antenatal period and continue through childhood and adolescence.

Services for children and young people

The Labour government manifesto has committed to improving access to clinically proven and cost-effective psychological therapies, acknowledging that current provision is too patchy whilst waiting times are too long (John-

Table 7.6 Vision from the NSF for children, young people and maternity services (DH, DfES, 2004c).

Government wants to see:

- An *improvement* in the mental health of all children and young people.
- That multi-agency services, working in partnership, *promote the mental health of all children and young people, provide early intervention* and also meet the needs of children and young people with established or complex problems.
- That all children, young people and their families have *access to mental health care based upon the best available evidence and provided by staff with an appropriate range of skills and competencies.*
- Improving services for 16- and 17-year-olds and those with learning disabilities.

son, 2007). Patel *et al.* (2007) propose a population-based, youth-focused, model of integrating mental health workers with youth health workers and welfare expertise. Those agencies involved in the professional support, advice and treatment of emotional and mental health problems need to be skilled, knowledgeable and confident. Services may be involved in helping children and young people, supporting their parents and family or supporting children and young people who have parents suffering mental ill health.

The National Service Framework for Children, Young People and their Families (DH/DfES, 2004c) has set national standards for the provision of care, and Standard 9 looks specifically at mental health services. The standard states that:

All children and young people, from birth to their eighteenth birthday, who have mental health problems and disorders have access to timely, integrated, high quality, multi-disciplinary mental health services to ensure effective assessment, treatment and support, for them and their families (NSF Standard 9: DH/DfES, 2004c).

The vision from government can be seen in Table 7.6.

Child and Adolescent Mental Health Services

The CAMHS tiered approach was developed in 1995 after a review of children's mental health (Health Advisory Service, 1995). This remains the approach advocated in subsequent policy (DH, 2001; DfEE, 2001; DH/DfES, 2004b,c,d) and has three main functions:

- Assessment and treatment
- Advice, support and consultation
- Promotion of mental health

Tier 1 is delivered by primary care practitioners (including school nurses, health visitors and other community nurses), GPs, social care practitioners and some educational professionals. All should have been trained to promote mental health, identify problems, offer advice and support and refer on to Tier 2 services if appropriate. This tier should ensure that minor (and sometimes more complex) issues are addressed early and effectively or managed safely until they can be seen by Tier 2 professionals.

Tier 2 work is provided by specialist CAMHS professionals such as educational psychologists, clinical psychologists, and community psychiatric nurses. However, there are also a large number of school nurses, health visitors and other community nurses and who may have undergone extra training to deal with problems at this level. It is also not uncommon to hear practitioners who are working at this level state that they are doing so without the training or support, due to lack of resources and long waiting lists in CAMHS.

Tier 3 and 4 services offer specialist services for severe and enduring mental illness. These specialist professionals should also provide training and consultation to other professionals.

This tiered approach should ensure that the responsiveness, accessibility and effectiveness of assessment and treatment are met through a range of services and professionals working together to meet the demand. The following are vital in this tiered provision of care:

- Provision of a comprehensive CAMHS
- Clear structures in place to facilitate referrals between the tiers
- Acknowledgement that CAMHS is everybody's business
- Education on promoting emotional well-being
- Improved access to services through expanded capacity and better skill mix

The government policy tabled above advocates collaborative working with children and families as being vital to the success of reducing the impact of mental ill health. There is evidence in the literature of collaboration between school, learning mentors, school nurses and CAMHS and also with health visitors, utilising solution-focused treatments (Walker and Townsend, 1998; Window *et al.*, 2004, Worral-Davies *et al.*, 2004). There is also more anecdotal evidence which has not been published and therefore the evidence base is not complete (DeBell and Tomkins, 2006). There is advice in the literature of the benefits of using one's self as a therapeutic tool when managing clients' mental health problems (Freshwater, 2002).

Use of self as a therapeutic tool

Freshwater (2002) suggests that the establishment of a therapeutic healing association attempts to redress the power balance, developing a close relationship so that care is planned in partnership. This requires from the 'professional' an awareness of self – revealing the real self versus the professional self. Freshwater (2002) argues that a truly healthy person is able to share some of their self with the client; promoting and maintaining one's own self-esteem will help support others to build theirs. In order to encourage the client to tell their story the 'professional' also requires excellent communication skills, including active and reflective listening and empathic awareness and catharsis. It is important, however, that practitioners understand the limitations of their role. Being aware of risk factors, protective factors and influences on mental health will also help them to deliver effective mental health promotion services.

Risk factors, protective factors and resilience

Some children and young people, in spite of traumatic events occurring in their life will cope without detrimental impact upon their mental health and well-being. Townley (2002) calls this resilience and suggests that protective factors are an easy temperament, higher intelligence and self-esteem, a supportive family and religion, and this is reiterated along with guidance on its promotion in policy documentation (DH, DfES, 2004b). Strochschein (2005) studied the effects of parental divorce on children and young people and provides insight into the vulnerability it causes in some children and young people such as anxiety, depression and anti-social behaviour, whilst others showed resilience in the face of this adversity.

Table 7.7 summarizes the features of resilient children and young people linked to their individual characteristics and the family influences upon them.

Frieson (2007) suggests that strategies aimed at improving parenting include attention to environmental factors such as family poverty, school, community and neighbourhood circumstances, and attention to policy. Specific training or support for parenting can also strengthen and increase children's adaptive capacity. Brooks's (2007) review of the literature on resilience provides useful guidance for minimising risks and promoting positive outcomes for children and young people and provides a rationale for strengthening the structure for resilience-building efforts in schools. Strategies such as developing social competence, increasing bonding between students and caring adults, communi-

Table 7.7 Resilience factors (Masten and Coatsworth, 1998; cited in Friesen, 2007).

Individual characteristics	**Family resources**
■ Good intellectual function	■ Close relationship to caring parent figure authoritative parenting
■ Easygoing disposition	
■ Self-efficacy	
■ Self-confidence	■ Warmth and structure
■ Talents	■ High expectations
	■ Socioeconomic advantages
	■ Connections to extended family networks

cating high expectations for students' academic and social performance and maximising opportunities for meaningful participation of students in the school environment are advocated (Brooks, 2007). There is debate in Frieson (2007) on risk and responsibility and its role in developing resilience which is beyond the scope of this chapter, but nevertheless very interesting.

Supporting children of parents with mental illness

Carers play a vital role in providing support for mental health service users and Standard 6 of the Mental Health NSF (DH, 1999) specifically addresses the needs of carers. It advocates that carers should have an annual assessment of their own mental health needs as the strains and responsibilities of caring can have an impact on mental and physical well-being (DH, 1999). What is not acknowledged in here is the impact upon the children of adults with mental illness. The government has produced guidance on *Developing Services for Carers and Families of People with Mental Illness* (DH, 2002) and this acknowledges children as carers and proposes the need for interventions to help support the whole family and promotes the parenting role of adults in the family as being more helpful for the child's welfare.

It is vital that children and young people who are supporting or living with parents with a mental illness are identified and offered support. The Children's Society has a database of young carers projects from around the country which are supporting children, young people and their families. Frank (2002) offers a good practice guide which aims to provide an evidence base for successful interventions and advocates multi-agency partnerships with children and young people at the centre.

Promoting own mental health

In order to deliver effective mental health promotion and effectively support those vulnerable to mental ill health, it is beneficial for those involved to be mentally healthy themselves. Undoubtedly the effect of managing mental ill health or distress in others impacts upon professionals' own personal well-being. Recognising what self and colleagues need to do to remain healthy and what they need from others to support them is important and this is a reflection on how much mental health is promoted within practice – individually and as a team. Clinical supervision from a skilled mental health professional is seen as advantageous and good practice (Walker and Townsend, 1998; Window *et al.*, 2004; Nursing and Midwifery Council, 2007). However, there are things that individuals can do such as valuing self, with time out for reflection and relaxation; talking issues and experiences through with others; and receiving supervision and guidance. Being able to provide a listening and empathic ear to each other will help ease the stress that dealing with mental health distress in others can cause.

Conclusion

It is important that parents and all professionals are supported to utilise all opportunities available to promote mental health and well-being in children and young people by building their confidence and self-esteem. Providing

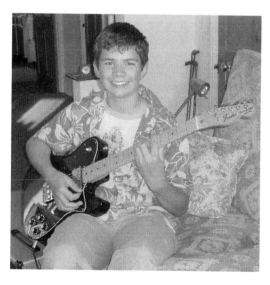

Learning a skill gives a sense of achievement

children and young people with supportive feedback will promote successful learning and being enabled to recognise their rights and resolve issues with respect will be skills that will have impact upon their adult lives too. It is vital that there is easy and early access to services when tensions and issues arise. If children and young people are to achieve their full potential and contribute successfully to the nation's growth and economy it is imperative that this essential aspect of health be delivered effectively.

Multi-agency education programmes which deliver effective development of knowledge, skills and confidence in mental health promotion and support will address needs effectively and appropriately and promote mental health. This requires:

- Education and training from appropriate experts
- Strategies to provide assessment and treatment
- Support for all from appropriate professionals
- A clear understanding of what being 'mentally healthy' means
- Knowledge in the difference between problems and disorders
- Awareness of risk factors, protective factors and influences on mental health
- Strategies for delivering effective mental health promotion

References

Acheson, Sir Donald (1998) *Independent Inquiry into Inequalities in Health.* http://www.official-documents.co.uk/document/doh/ih/ih.htm; accessed November 2003.

Ahmad, Y., Dalrymple, J., Daum, M., Griffiths, N., Hockridge, T. and Ryan, E. (2003) *Listening to Children and Young People.* University of West of England, Bristol.

Barnes, J. (2005) 'You could see it on their faces...': The importance of provoking smiles in schools. *Health Education*, **105**(5), 392–400.

Brooks, J. E. (2006) Strengthening resilience in children and youths: maximizing opportunities through the schools. *Children & Schools*, **28**(2), 69–76.

Child Mental Health Centre (2007) http://www.childmentalhealthcentre.org/; accessed 5 January 2008.

DeBell, D. and Tomkins, A. S. (2006) *Discovering the Future of School Nursing: the Evidence Base.* CPHVA, London.

Department for Education and Skills (2004) *Healthy Living Blueprint.* DfES, London.

Department Of Health (1999) *National Service Framework for Mental Health.* http://www.nsfmentalhealth.gov.uk/; accessed April 2004.

Department Of Health (1999a) *Saving Lives – Our Healthier Nation.* Stationery Office, London.

Department of Health (1999b) *Making a Difference: Strengthening the Nursing, Midwifery and Health Visiting Contributions to Health and Healthcare.* Stationery Office, London.

Department of Health (2000) *The NHS Plan: A Plan for Investment. A Plan for Reform.* Stationery Office, London.

Department of Health (2001) *The Journey to Recovery – The Government's Vision of Mental Health Care.* Department of Health, London.

Department of Health (2001b) *Health Visitor Practice Development Resource Pack.* Stationery Office, London.

Department of Health (2002) *Developing Services for Carers and Families of People with Mental Illness.* DH, London.

Department of Health (2004a) *Choosing Health. Making Healthier Choices Easier.* Stationery Office, London.

Department of Health (2004b) *The Chief Nursing Officer's Review of the Nursing, Midwifery and Health Visiting Contribution to Vulnerable Children and Young People.* Department of Health, London.

Department of Health (2006) *School Nurse Practice Development Resource Pack.* Stationery Office, London.

Department of Health (2007) *Children, Families and Maternity E-bulletin – Sept 2007.* Gateway 8745.

Department of Health & Community Practitioners' and Health Visitors' Association (2003) *Liberating the Public Health Talents of Community Practitioners and Health Visitors.* Stationery Office, London.

Department of Health and the Department for Education and Employment (1999) *The National Healthy Schools Standard.* DfEE, London.

Department of Health and Department for Education and Skills (2003) *Every Child Matters.* http://www.everychildmatters.gov.uk/; accessed 20 June 2007.

Department Of Health and Department for Education and Skills (2004a) *National Healthy Schools Programme.* DfES: London. http://www.wiredforhealth.gov.uk/.

Department Of Health and Department for Education and Skills (2004b) *Promoting Emotional Health and Well-Being Through the National Healthy School Standard.* DfES: London. http://www.wiredforhealth.gov.uk/.

Department of Health and Department for Education and Skills (2004c) *National Service Framework for Children, Young People and Maternity Services.* http://www. dh.gov.uk/publicationspolicy/.

Department of Health and Department for Education and Skills (2004d) *Every Child Matters – The Next Steps.* Stationery Office, London.

Department for Education and Employment (2001) *Promoting Children's Mental Health within Early Years and School Settings.* DfEE, London.

Derisley, J., Libby, S., Clark, S. and Reynolds, S. (2005) Mental health, coping and family functioning in parents of young people with obsessive-compulsive disorder and with anxiety disorders. *British Journal of Clinical Psychology*, **44**, 439–44.

Favazza, A. R. (1996) *Bodies Under Siege: Self Mutilation and Body Modification in Culture and Psychiatry*, 2nd edn. Johns Hopkins Press, Baltimore.

Frank, J. (2002) *Making it Work: Good Practice with Young Carers and Their Families.* http://www.childrenssociety.org.uk/; accessed 28 September 2007.

Frieson, B. J. (2007) Recovery and resilience in children's mental health: views from the field. *Psychiatric Rehabilitation Journal*, **31**(1), 38–48.

Freshwater, D. (2002) *Therapeutic Nursing – Improving Patient Care Through Self Awareness and Reflection.* Sage, London.

Geller, D. A., Biederman, J., Jones, J., Shapiro, S., Schwartz, S. and Park, K. S. (1998) Obsessive compulsive disorder in children and adolescents: a review. *Harvard Review of Psychiatry*, **5**, 260–73.

Health Advisory Service (1995) *Together We Stand: Child and Adolescent Mental Health Services*. HMSO, London.

Johnson, A. (2007) *Speech to the House of Commons 12/9/07*. http://www.dh.gov.uk/en/News/Speeches/DH_078397; accessed 14 September 2007.

The Mental Health Foundation (2007a) *Depression*. http://www.mentalhealth.org.uk/information/mental-health-a-z/depression/; accessed 29 September 2007.

The Mental Health Foundation (2007b) *Eating Disorders*. http://www.mentalhealth.org.uk/information/mental-health-a-z/eating-disorders/; accessed 29 September 2007.

The Mental Health Foundation (2007c) *Self Harm*. http://www.mentalhealth.org.uk/; accessed on 12 September 2007.

National Institute for Mental Health in England (2007) *Inside Outside: Improving Mental Health Services for Black and Minority Ethnic Communities in England*. DH, London.

National Institute for Health and Clinical Excellence (2004a) *Eating Disorders: Core Interventions in the Treatment and Management of Anorexia Nervosa, Bulimia Nervosa and Related Eating Disorders*. NICE Clinical Guideline No. 9. Available from http://www.nice.org.uk/CG009/.

National Institute for Health and Clinical Excellence (2004b) *Self Harm: the Short Term Physical and Secondary Prevention of Self Harm in Primary and Secondary Care*. NICE Clinical Guideline No. 16. Available from http://www.nice.org.uk/CG016/.

National Institute for Health and Clinical Excellence (2004c) *Anxiety: Management of Anxiety (Panic Disorder, with or Without Agoraphobia, and Generalized Anxiety Disorder) in Adults in Primary, Secondary and Community Care*. NICE Clinical Guideline No. 22. Available from http://www.nice.org.uk/CG022/.

National Institute for Health and Clinical Excellence (2005) *Depression in Children and Young People: Identification and Management in Primary, Community and Secondary Care*. NICE Clinical Guideline No. 28. Available from http://www.nice.org.uk/CG028NICEguideline/.

Nursing and Midwifery Council (2007) *Clinical Supervision Advice Sheet*. http://www.nmc-uk.org/aFrameDisplay.aspx?DocumentID=1558; accessed 29 September 2007).

Patel, V., Flisher, A. J., Hetrick, S. and McGorry, P. (2007) Mental health of young people: a global challenge. *Lancet*, **14**(369), 1302–13.

Preece, P. and Jowett, S. (2007) Why do young people self-harm? *British Journal of School Nursing*, **2**(1), 20–3.

Sainsbury Centre for Mental Health (2007) *Feeling Good: Promoting Children's Mental Health*. http://www.scmh.org.uk/; accessed 28 August 2007.

Salkovskis, P., Shafron, R., Rachman, S. and Freeston, M. H. (1999) Multiple pathways to inflated responsibility beliefs in obsessional problems: Possible origins and implications for therapy and research. *Behaviour Research and Therapy*, **37**, 1055–72.

Souter, A. and Kramer, S. (2004) 'Given up hope of dying': A child protection approach to deliberate self harm in adolescents admitted to a paediatric ward. *Child and Family Social Work*, **9**, 259–64.

Strohschein, L. (2005) Parental divorce and child mental health trajectories. *Journal of Marriage and Family*, **67**(5), 1286–300.

Townley, M. (2002) Mental health needs of children and young people. *Nursing Standard* **16**(30), 38–45.

United Nations Children's Fund [UNICEF] (2007) *Child Poverty in Perspective: an Overview of Child Well-being in Rich Countries*. Innocenti Report Card 7. Innocenti Research Centre, Florence.

Vimpani, G. (2005) Getting the mix right: family, community and social policy interventions to improve outcomes for young people at risk of substance misuse. *Drug and Alcohol Review*, **24**(2), 111–25.

Walker, Z. and Townsend, J. (1998) Promoting adolescent mental health in primary care: a review of the literature. *Journal of Adolescence*, **21**, 621–34.

Wanless, Sir D. (2004) *Securing Good Health for the Whole Population*. http://www.hm-treasury.gov.uk/media/32287/wanless_health_trends.pdf

Window, S., Anderson, L. and Vostanis, P. (2004) A multi-agency service for child behavioural problems. *Community Practitioner*, **77**(5), 180–4.

Whooley, M. A., Avins, A. L., Miranda, J. and Browner, W. S. (1997) Case-finding instruments for depression. Two questions are as good as many. *J. Gen. Intern. Med.*, **12**(7), 439–45.

Wolpert, M., Fuggle, P., Cottrell, D., Fonagy, P., Phillips, J., Pilling, S., Stein, S. and Target, M. (2006) *Drawing on the Evidence: Advice for Mental Health Professionals Working with Children and Adolescents*, 2nd edn. CAMHS Publications, London.

Worrall-Davies, A., Cottrell, D. and Benson, E. (2004) Evaluation of an early intervention Tier 2 child and adolescent mental health service. *Health and Social Care in the Community*, **12**(2), 119–25.

Young Minds (2006) *Facts and Figures*. http://www.youngminds.org.uk/problems/facts_0.php; accessed 30 June 2006.

Young Minds (2007) *Problems*. http://www.youngminds.org.uk/problems/links.php; accessed 2 September 2007.

Young Minds (2007) *Eating Disorders*. http://www.youngminds.org.uk/eatingproblems/index.php; accessed 29 September 2007.

Useful websites

Child Mental Health Centre: http://www.childmentalhealthcentre.org/

Children's Society Young Carer's Initiative: http://www.youngcarer.com/showPage.php?file=index.htm

http://www.rcpsych.ac.uk/info/mhgu/newmhgu14.htm

http://www.bullying.co.uk/

The Mental Health Foundation: http://www.mentalhealth.org.uk/

Audit Commission: http://www.audit-commission.gov.uk/

Young Minds: http://www.youngminds.org.uk/

CHAPTER 8

Sexual health within the public health agenda

Pat Day

Key themes

- Sexual health as a public health priority
- Adolescent sexual health
- The delivery of teenage sexual health services

Case study

In 2007, a 15-year-old attended a busy young people's sexual health clinic with her friends. She had been shopping and thought that she would pop in. When asked why she had come, a casual remark indicated that her period was late. A positive pregnancy test and scan revealed that she was 19 weeks pregnant. She was incredulous that she had become pregnant and asked for a termination. Displaying little emotion about her predicament, she was adamant she could not tell her mother because she would 'kill her'. The implications of a late termination slowly dawned on her. The trauma of this experience affected not only this young woman and her family but also the staff who cared for her. The prevention of such traumatic events is the subject of this chapter.

Introduction

Increasing priority has been given to young people's sexual health by the government (Department of Health [DH], 2001; DH, 2004a; Department for

Education and Skills [DfES/DH], 2006). However, rates of unplanned teenage pregnancy and sexually transmitted infections remain unacceptably high (NICE, 2007). There has been a gradual shift towards recognising the contribution that school nurses can make to the public health agenda (DH, 1999a,b, 2001). The present climate offers primary care workers the opportunity to make a real difference to young people's sexual health. They are now in a pivotal position to contribute to multi agency efforts to resolve the adolescent sexual health crisis. Through understanding the determinants of teenage sexual behaviour and the evidence base for effective interventions, they can translate government rhetoric into action and lead innovative interventions which could improve adult sexual health.

The current situation

The aphorism that there are 'lies, damned lies and statistics' could be applied to teenage sexual health. Rates of teenage pregnancy are reported as the lowest for twenty years (Teenage Pregnancy Unit, 2007). Under 18 and under 16 conception rates have fallen by 11.8% and 12.1% since 1998. On the face of it this seems a real achievement and should be celebrated. However, it is important to examine the implications for practice of this reported decrease.

There were still 39,683 conceptions to under 18s in 2005 (Table 8.1). The reduction from 46.6 to 41.1 conceptions per thousand is encouraging but still remains high. These national statistics must also be examined in line with local

Table 8.1 Under 18 conceptions for England: 1998–2005 (Office for National Statistics, 2007).

Year	Number of under 18 conceptions	Under 18 conception rate*	Percentage leading to legal abortion
1998	41,089	46.6	42.4
1999	39,247	44.8	43.5
2000	38,699	43.6	44.8
2001	38,461	42.5	46.1
2002	39,350	42.6	45.8
2003	39,553	42.1	46.1
2004	39,593	41.5	46.0
2005**	39,683	41.1	46.9

*per thousand females aged 15–17
**provisional

statistics, which often reveal a different picture. In Sheffield, there has been an increase from 1998 of 431 conceptions in under 18s to 477 in 2005 (Teenage Pregnancy Unit, 2007).

Under 16 conceptions

The provisional under 16 conception rate for England in 2005 was 7.8 per 1000 girls aged 13–15 (Table 8.2). This is 12.1% lower than the Teenage Pregnancy Strategy's 1998 baseline rate of 8.8 conceptions per 1000 girls aged 13–15.

Under 16 conceptions should be a cause of even greater concern. They can cause long-lasting damage to the health of adolescents (Mayor, 2004). The reduction in the number of these pregnancies is disappointing. There has also been a sharp increase from 2004 to 2005 and this requires close scrutiny. Specialist community public health nurses need to become adept at interpreting government statistics and should approach them with caution. They often do not represent the whole picture. Health need should be assessed on a combination of national and local agendas. This involves exercising the skills of a public health practitioner and looking in depth at the reality of a situation (DfES/DH, 2006).

A decrease in teenage pregnancy does not correlate with the startling increase in sexually transmitted infections amongst the young (Health Protection Agency [HPA], 2005) (Figure 8.1). Adolescents are disproportionately represented in the sharply accelerating rate of sexually transmitted infections. Rates of chlamydia, gonorrhoea, genital warts and genital herpes are steadily

Table 8.2 Under 16 conceptions for England: 1998–2005 (Office for National Statistics, 2007; Teenage Pregnancy Unit, 2007).

Year	Under 16 conceptions	Under 16 conception rate*	Percentage leading to legal abortion
1998	7,855	8.8	52.9
1999	7,408	8.2	53.0
2000	7,620	8.3	54.5
2001	7,407	8.0	56.0
2002	7,395	7.9	55.7
2003	7,558	7.9	57.6
2004	7,181	7.5	57.6
2005**	7,462	7.8	57.4

*per thousand females aged 13–15
**provisional

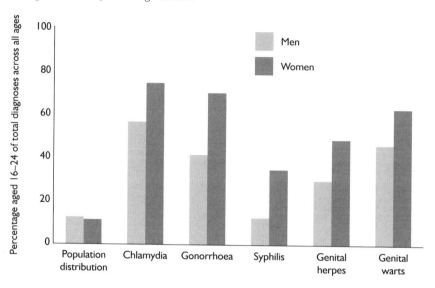

Figure 8.1 The rate of STIs in 16–24 year olds.

increasing among 16 to 24-year-olds (HPA, 2005). Sexual infections can cause permanent damage to health (DH, 2001) and chlamydia is the most common sexually transmitted infection amongst the young. Between 2000 and 2004 diagnoses of chlamydia increased by 56% in 16 to 19-year-old females. Corresponding statistics for males are not provided (HPA, 2005). Young women aged 16 to 24 make up 74% and 56% respectively of all chlamydia diagnoses. Undiagnosed chlamydia may result in pelvic inflammatory disease, infertility and ectopic pregnancy (Moens *et al.*, 2003). Genital herpes is a lifelong condition which can cause long-term physical and psychological pain (Lebrun-Vignes *et al.*, 2007).

The genital wart virus is associated with cervical cancer (Rambout *et al.*, 2007). Human papilloma virus is the wart virus which causes invasive cervical cancer (DH, 2007). In 2008, the government announced that the HPV vaccine will be offered to all 12 to 13-year-old girls. This is a major step forward for women's health. Recommendations are that this will be delivered in schools (DH, 2007). Although mass immunisation campaigns impact on school nurse activity, public health nurses have a responsibility to facilitate programmes which have measurable health outcomes. The HPV vaccine will prevent 70% of infections by the wart virus (DH, 2007). However, it is important to guard against complacency as the results of the vaccination programme will not be seen immediately. In response to this serious public health issue, school nurses should ensure that initiatives pay as much attention to the prevention of sexually transmitted infections as pregnancy.

Behind the statistics

Poverty is a strong determinant of poor teenage sexual health (NICE, 2007). Deprived communities have the highest rates of teenage pregnancy (DfES, 2006). This compounds social and economic disadvantage. The impact of teenage pregnancy means that there has been emphasis on examining its causes and consequences. However, it remains a complex and elusive issue. When teenage girls are asked why they became pregnant, they often cannot give an answer.

There is a pattern in the characteristics of adolescent parents. Low attainment, disliking school and non-attendance at school are important factors (DfES, 2006). 60% of boys and 47% of girls who leave school with no qualifications had sex before they were 16. They are also much less likely to use contraception than peers who have qualifications. School nurses have a vital role to play in multi-agency efforts to raise attainment in poorly achieving schools. This can be seen as part of their remit within the healthy schools initiative (DfES/DH, 2006).

Other social determinants include being looked after, having a teenage mother or coming from a black ethnic background (DfES, 2006). There may be an argument for school nurses to discriminate positively in favour of these groups. Interventions should be targeted to the needs of vulnerable groups and take account of social and cultural background.

The impact of the statistics

The negative impact of teenage pregnancy has resulted in it becoming a priority target. It severely affects the outcomes of mothers and babies (DfES, 2006). Young women are unlikely to complete their education and are often destined to bring up their child alone and in poverty. They are more likely to smoke during pregnancy and bottle feed their babies. Their mental health is often poor, with a much higher incidence of post-natal depression than older mothers (DfES, 2006). Infant mortality is 60% greater in this age group (DfES, 2006).

It makes economic sense to concentrate strategies on preventing teenage pregnancy. The cost to the NHS is estimated at £63 million a year and benefit payments can add astronomically to this bill (DfES, 2006). School nurses have a responsibility to dedicate time and energy to the needs of this group. Efforts should be directed towards primary prevention of unplanned teenage pregnancy. However, this should not mean that the needs of teenage mothers are neglected. Many of these young women are lost to the school nursing service when they become pregnant. It could be argued that this vulnerable population requires the services of dedicated school nurses.

Case study

This model has been successfully adopted by the school nursing service in Doncaster (Doncaster PCT, 2007). Through the appointment of a specialist school nurse for young people not in mainstream education, young mothers in a teenage pregnancy unit are able to access education and services. As many of them have missed out on their education, the school nurse provides one-to-one support. A comprehensive health education package is also delivered in the classroom. Whilst these young women are able to obtain contraception through an outreach sexual health nurse, they are also supported in attending mainstream services. Some of these clients now feel confident enough to access services on their own. The project is in the early stage of development, but preliminary results are showing promising outcomes and could provide a model for future service delivery.

The determinants of teenage sexual health

Adolescence is a critical time in a person's lifespan. This period is marked by a search for identity (Erikson, 1970). Exploration of roles can lead to confusion and uncertainty. High levels of risk-taking and health-compromising behaviour can characterise this stage of development (Barron, 2005). Adolescents are naturally egocentric (Piaget, 1972) and they indulge in 'magical thinking' (White, 1987). This means that they can see that certain actions may harm others, but they regard themselves as invincible and cannot accept that they could be harmed. In a world largely unsupported by adults, this is a recipe for disaster.

Boys and girls are reaching puberty earlier (McCarney and Hendee, 1989) and having sex younger (Wellings *et al* 1994). Early sex is more common in girls who were under 13 at puberty (Wellings *et al.*, 2001). One in three under 16-year-olds are reported as being sexually active (Paton, 2002).

Creation of a modern society

Being sexually active at a young age is associated with an increased number of sexual partners (Cribier *et al.*, 1996) and less use of contraception (Mahoney, 2000; Wright, 1999). These are important indicators for school nurses. Girls as young as 9 are experiencing puberty and they require age-appropriate sex education to equip them with the knowledge to deal with the physical and emotional impact. School nurses can influence the delivery of sex education by presenting the evidence base in favour of early education. This includes the consideration of sex education programmes which advocate 'delayed sex'.

Parents are an important factor in shaping adolescent behaviour. A lack of parental supervision is associated with greater risk taking behaviours (Whaley *et al.*, 1999). In a tracking survey for the Teenage Pregnancy Strategy, half of young people said their parents gave them very little information about sex (BMRB International, 2003). Rates of contraceptive use are higher in young men whose parents discuss sex positively (Stone and Ingham, 2002). However, fathers are particularly bad at talking about sex with their children (BMRB International, 2003). This has implications for the sexual health of boys. A successful project has been running in Sheffield for ten years which trains parents to talk to their children about sex (Sheffield Centre for HIV and Sexual Health, 2007). The Parent-to-Parent project has helped over 1,000 parents in the city. It has been recognised by the government as an example of good practice. Support for parents has been recognised within the public health remit of the school nurse (DfES/DH, 2006) and it should be integrated into all initiatives to improve adolescent health.

In their move to independence, adolescents withdraw from parents and move closer to their peers. Teenagers who mix with sexually active peers are more likely to have sex earlier themselves (Weyman, 2003). An awareness of this risk factor means that this group requires more education and communication from health professionals. British teenagers live in a highly sexualised society, but are not encouraged to discuss the implications of this with adults (Weyman, 2003). Ambivalent attitudes to young people and their sexual health results in them receiving mixed messages. The media suggest that sexual activity is the norm and to be encouraged (Hausser and Michaud, 1994). Until recently little responsibility has been attached to media portrayal of sexual relationships and discussion of contraception in films or television has been minimal (Kelly, 2001). This encourages a *laissez faire* attitude to its use. However, television soap operas have begun to tackle these issues responsibly. In *EastEnders*, Demi Miller was 13 when she gave birth to her daughter Aleesha Beyonce. This storyline offered scope for discussing the difficulties of being a young teenage mother. Leo, Aleesha's father, also suffers rejection by his family and dies of a drug overdose. The media can contribute to conveying the realities of being a young parent.

Adopting a public health approach to sexual health promotion involves assessing and targeting the needs of teenagers. Understanding the world from their point of view means that interventions are more likely to be teenage-friendly and therefore effective.

Sex education

Case study

In 1996 two school nurses in Sheffield responded to the high rate of teenage pregnancies in an inner city comprehensive school by contributing to sex education classes. This was considered quite revolutionary at the time and involved overcoming the barriers to explicit sex education in the classroom. During lessons explicit information was given about contraception, including practical instructions about how to use condoms. The 'carrot' lessons, as they became known, were very popular and attracted media attention. They were filmed by Channel 4 for a programme about sex from 8 to 18 (Channel 4, 1999). They apparently contributed to a drop in teenage pregnancy in one comprehensive, although this was impossible to prove.

However, when developing sex education lessons, it became apparent that knowledge was only part of the key to tackling teenage sexual health. Knowledge of contraception does not predict actual use (van den Akker *et al.*, 1999). Teenagers know that they should use condoms but find it difficult to negotiate their use. The relationship between knowledge of contraception and sexual behaviour is complex and should be considered in both classroom education and one-to-one consultations.

Simply imparting information does not change behaviour (Stephenson *et al.*, 2003). Strong evidence supports school-based education, particularly when linked to contraceptive services (Swann *et al.*, 2003). The components of successful programmes are not entirely clear, but appear to include a theoretical basis and be targeted to need (Ellis and Grey, 2004). School-based interventions based on socio-cognitive theories such as theory of reasoned action (Fishbein and Ajzen, 1975) and social learning theory (Bandura, 1986) are much more likely to be effective than those that are not (Fishbein, 2000).

Characteristics of effective programmes include complex activities which require time and commitment (Kirby, 2001). These include education to resist social pressure, communication and assertiveness training. Materials and teaching methods should match the group. The Dutch model of sex education is based on this approach. It has a focus on relationship and communication skills (Valk, 2000). It is also research-based and benefits from well-resourced central dissemination of information.

Case study

A travel scholarship enabled two British health workers to visit Dutch schools and observe their programme in action. It was evident that Dutch teachers had a more informal relationship with students and were more willing to disclose their own feelings about relationships (Day and Lane, 1999). A video made by a Dutch teacher showed teachers recounting their first sexual encounters, including the admission by one teacher that he was gay. Teachers in Holland can give confidential advice to pupils without fear of reprisal. This leads to explicit exchanges of information and discussion of taboo subjects such as homosexuality. The legal and cultural differences between the Netherlands and Britain mean that there are limits to what would be acceptable in British schools. However, there are lessons that can be drawn about greater openness and honesty when discussing sex with young people.

The Dutch use drama to explore the complexities within adolescent sexual relationships. A drama production called 'Stepping over the mark' was performed in a secondary school in a deprived suburb of Rotterdam. It was written and produced by students (Day and Lane, 1999). This was about girls being persuaded to have sex by their boyfriends. The audience was mesmerised by the performances of their peers.

The Dutch have adopted a pragmatic approach to teenage sex. They appreciate and value youth. Their message to the young about safe sex is unambiguous and backed up by easy access to contraception.

The national situation

In a survey by *CosmoGirl* magazine, one third of teenagers thought their sex and relationships education (SRE) was 'rubbish' and 81% thought that it could be improved (Smith, 2006). Guidelines for sex education in schools remain vague and open to interpretation. It is a statutory requirement for schools to provide sex and relationships education (DfEE, 1996). The national curriculum for science includes the biology of sex. Apart from this, there are no clear directives about what should be included or how it should be delivered. As a result, provision is patchy – too concentrated on information giving and lacking in evaluation (Ofsted, 2002). Levels of education are not considered adequate to prepare young people for life in a complex society (UNICEF, 2001). Parents can withdraw children from the SRE programme. This does not happen in the Netherlands and could be considered a violation of the rights of the child. There is also an emphasis on marriage which does not fit with an inclusive view of what constitutes a family (DfEE, 2000).

Lack of specific direction has had a negative impact on sex education in primary schools. This is often squeezed into the curriculum after SATs and between summer drama productions and sports days. When 16-year-olds were asked about sex education, they said that they needed it 'earlier on' (Bourton, 2006, p. 21). They also felt that it should be accurate and detailed because this would discourage experimentation. 'If you know all about it, I mean real details, then you would be happier to wait. But because it is such a "hush hush" subject the mystery makes you curious' (Bourton, 2006, p. 24). Sex education should begin at the age of five and be delivered through a spiral curriculum.

Successful approaches to sex education

The most effective sex education programmes are multi-faceted and involve a joint agency approach (DiCenso *et al.*, 2002). They are delivered over time, offer consistent messages and emphasise communication (Thistle and Ray, 2002). School nurses can play a pivotal role in contributing to these programmes. They offer a confidential, objective and knowledgeable service which should complement the role of teachers (Thistle and Ray, 2002). Teachers are bound by different codes of professional conduct and have a duty to inform the head teacher if a student discloses under-age sexual activity (Department for Education, 1994). Drawing on the strengths of different disciplines is a characteristic of the best programmes. School nurses and teachers should work together in the classroom to convey clear information and messages. The demarcation lines in professional responsibilities should be explained to students in order to avoid confusion.

The most promising interventions embrace both a behavioural component and a multi-agency delivery. They include the APAUSE (added Power and Understanding in Sex Education) SRE programme which has been developed by the University of Exeter (Blenkinsop *et al.*, 2004). It has incorporated a spiral approach to health promotion with curriculum materials for Years 7 and

8, sessions in Years 9 and 10 led by teachers and health professionals, and an evaluation questionnaire in Year 11. A spiral curriculum begins with simple concepts and then builds on this foundation with more complex information and ideas. It is considered good practice in an education system which values discovery learning.

Joint training is also the gold standard for the delivery of sex education programmes. It is difficult to achieve and requires additional resources. This is one of the strengths of the APAUSE programme. Training is delivered to teachers and health professionals by an external coordinator. This ensures a consistent approach to delivery. Handbooks are provided with scripted materials. There is an emphasis on story-telling to relay key messages. APAUSE has a strong peer-led component in year nine. This is seen as innovative and effective (Blenkinsop *et al.*, 2004).

Evaluation of APAUSE has shown a small but significant difference in terms of reported sexual activity (Blenkinsop *et al.*, 2004). Students who had undertaken the programme were less likely to be sexually active than comparison students. If they had sex, they were more likely to have used contraception. The problem with the APAUSE programme is its poor dissemination. Many authorities are prohibited from using it due to its cost. Shortage of school nurses was also highlighted as an issue in its evaluation (Blenkinsop *et al.*, 2004). School nurses should be proactive in advocating for the widespread use of APAUSE due to its demonstrated effectiveness. Involvement in these programmes needs to be made a priority as it can make a real difference to the impact on teenagers.

Access to sexual health services

Whilst the ideal in preventative programmes is to delay sexual activity, the problem is that more young people are having sex younger and taking risks with their sexual health. The most effective way of preventing teenage pregnancy is to combine good sex education with local access to services (University of York, 1997). Teenagers have the same rights as adults to treatment and can give their own consent if they are considered Fraser competent (Gillick v. West Norfolk and Wisbech, 1985). However, young people perceive clinical services as judgemental, difficult to access and lacking in confidentiality (Barrister *et al.*, 2002). In response to an unmet need, the Teenage Pregnancy Unit has advocated for the development of young people's clinics which focus on at risk groups and are targeted to local need (Swann *et al.*, 2003).

Consultation with young people is vital in shaping services. It is one of the hallmarks of areas with the largest decreases in teenage pregnancy (Ingham *et al.*, 2000). Adolescents want confidential, accessible, frequent services with no appointments (Brook, 1998). They tend not to trust GPs (Peckham *et al.*, 1996). In response to this, some GPs have adopted a teenage-friendly model in their approach to young people. In South Gloucestershire surgeries are badged 'no worries' if staff have been trained and services designed with adolescents in mind (DfES/DH, 2005).

Other innovative interventions such as 'clinics in a box' are also showing promising results. In 2003–2004, 4,500 young people attended a mobile sexual health service in North Staffordshire (DH, 2004b); 47% of these clients were young men. The needs of young men are rarely addressed within mainstream services. Lessons can be learned from the development of male-only sexual health pilot projects in the Wirral and Derby (Hancock, 2004). These services are designed with boys in mind. Clients are seen quickly in an informal and respectful environment. Alongside these education projects, there is a need to develop clinical sites which are sensitive to male clients. An example of this is an outreach GUM clinic in London specifically for young men (Lewis *et al.*, 2004). This utilises an established Brook clinic site to target an inner city area where young men's sexual health is poor. Its success in reaching this population could serve as a model for future service delivery.

Case study

One of the first outreach services on a school site was set up in Sheffield (Lane and Day, 2001). This was in direct response to a request from teenage boys to 'gis some jonnies miss'. Collaboration took place with teachers, governors, the family planning service, local GPs and youth workers. It was decided to hold a Monday drop-in after school in a youth club. This was conveniently located in school grounds. Group work was conducted by a male youth worker and individual consultations were held with school nurses. The service provided condoms, emergency contraception and pregnancy tests. It was evident that many of the clients would not have attended central services. However, there were drawbacks to the proximity of the service to the school. Some young people complained that they were labelled as 'gay' by their peers. They resented being recognised as attending a sexual health service.

Despite its shortcomings, this model of service delivery was considered innovative and successful. It has been widely disseminated. Rigorous evaluation of this mode of service delivery is essential as the impact of these programmes is not clear (Swann *et al.*, 2003).

Future developments

Nurse prescribing offers school nurses the opportunity for further development of nurse led services. School nurses could advocate for emergency contraception and condoms to be included on the limited formulary (British Medical Association, 2006). An alternative to sexual health drop-ins may be the inclusion of a general service within an extended school. This could be less stigmatising and cover a wide range of health issues.

Screening for chlamydia should be integrated into the development of contraceptive services for young people. Pioneering work in York means that chlamydia testing is offered in 70% of secondary schools through sexual health drop ins (Taylor, 2006). Other areas have also taken up the mantle. In a school in Brighton, described as the 'chlamydia capital of Sussex', screening is offered through the Department of Health programme for under 25-year-olds (Taylor, 2006). An extension to this service could be the administration of treatment by school nurses. This may offer access to hard to reach groups within the school community.

Boys are difficult to engage with sexual health services. They are 'half the problem and half the solution' (Social Exclusion Unit, 1999). Little is known about what they want from services. They rarely attend clinics on their own and most of their information about sex comes from pornography (Wallmyr and Welin, 2006). There is a need for male workers to engage with boys and uncover their beliefs and attitudes.

The involvement of peer educators is popular with young people and requires further evaluation (Swann *et al.*, 2003). The training and availability of peer educators are important issues to consider. The influence of peers is powerful for teenagers and may make a difference to their decisions.

Conclusion

Adolescents make up 15% of the population (Metcalfe, 2004). The allocation of services to meet their needs does not reflect this statistic. School nurses with teachers, youth workers and others are in an ideal position to understand the determinants of their behaviour and influence the ways in which adolescent services are developed. Without increased resources and teenage-friendly services, adolescent sexual health will continue to deteriorate. There are profound inequalities in terms of funding for sexual health and youth services. As public health practitioners, school nurses have a responsibility to prioritise young people and their sexual health. If they do, the benefits for adult health are likely to last for generations.

References

Bandura, A. (1986) *Social Foundations of Thought and Action. A Social Cognitive Theory*. Prentice Hall, New Jersey.

Barrister, P., Fettiplace, R., Dolan, F., Massil, H. and Cowley, S. (2002) Quality, mainstream services with proactive and targeted outreach: a model of contraceptive service provision *Journal of Family Planning and Reproductive Health Care*, **28**(2), 90–4.

Barron, S. (2005) Sexual health of adolescents. *Primary Health Care*, **15**(5), 37–40.

Blenkinsop, S., Wade, P., Benton, T., Gnaldi, M. and Schagen, S. (2004) *Evaluation of the APAUSE Sex and Relationships Education Programme*. http://www.dfes.gov. uk/; accessed 14 November 2007.

BMRB International (2003) *Evaluation of the Teenage Pregnancy Strategy. Tracking Survey. Report of Results of Nine Waves of Research*. BMRB International, London. http://www.Teenagepregnancyunit.gov.uk/; accessed 24 August 2007.

Bourton, V. (2006) Sex education in schools: young people's views *Paediatric Nursing*, **18**(8), 20–4.

British Medical Association (2006) *BNF for Children*. BMJ Publishing Group, London.

Brook (1998) *'Someone with a Smile Would Be Your Best Bet...' What Young People Want From Sex Advice Centres*. Brook Advisory Centres, London.

Bruner, J. (1960) *The Process of Education*. Harvard University Press, Cambridge.

Cribier, B., Schmitt, M., Le Coz, C. and Grosshans, E. (1996) Changes in sexual behaviour of patients attending a HIV testing centre: a prospective study 1988–1994. *Genitourinary medicine*, **72**(2), 37–42.

Day, P. and Lane, D. (1999) Sex education: lessons to be learnt from going Dutch. *Community Practitioner*, **72**(8), 259–60.

Department for Education (1994) *Sex Education in Schools*. Circular number 5/94, Education Act 1993. HMSO, London.

Department for Education and Employment (1996) *Education Act*. HMSO, London.

Department for Education and Employment (2000) *Sex and Relationship Education Guidance*. DfEE, London.

Department for Education and Skills (2006) *Teenage Pregnancy Next Steps: Guidance for Local Authorities and Primary Care Trusts on Effective Delivery of Local Strategies*. DfES, Nottingham.

Department for Education and Skills and Department of Health (2005) *No Worries; Young People Friendly Badged Gps in North Somerset and Wiltshire*. http://www. everychildmatters.gov.uk/; accessed 14 November 2007.

Department of Health (1999a) *Saving Lives; Our Healthier Nation*. Stationery Office, London.

Department of Health (1999b) *Making a Difference: Strengthening the Nursing, Midwifery and Health Visiting Contribution to Health and Healthcare*. DH, London.

Department of Health (2001) *The National Strategy for Sexual Health and HIV*. DH, London.

Department of Health (2004a) *Choosing Health: Making Healthy Choices Easier*. Stationery Office, London.

Department of Health (2004b) Case Studies. http://www.childrensnsfcasestudies. dh.gov.uk/; accessed 14 November 2007.

Department of Health (2007) *HPV Vaccine Recommended for NHS Immunisation Programme*. http://www.gnn.gov.uk/; accessed 9 November 2007.

Department for Education and Skills/Department of Health (2006) *School Nurse: Practice Development Resource Pack*. DfES Publications, Nottingham.

DiCenso, A., Guyatt, G., Willan, A. and Griffith, L. (2002) Interventions to reduce unintended pregnancies among adolescents: systematic review of randomised controlled trials. *British Medical Journal*, **324**(7351), 1426–30.

Doncaster PCT (2007) *Targeted Interventions*. Unpublished.

Ellis, S. and Grey, A. (2004) NHS Development Agency *Prevention of Sexually Transmitted Infections: a Review of Reviews Into the Effectiveness of Non-clinical Interventions*. http://www.nice.org.uk/; accessed 24 August 2007.

Erikson, E. (1970) Reflections on the dissent of contemporary youth. *International Journal of Psychoanalysis*, **51**, 11–22.

Fishbein, M. and Ajzen, I. (1975) *Belief, Attitude, Intention and Behaviour: an Introduction to Theory and Research*. Addison-Wesley, Reading, MA.

Fishbein, M. (2000) The role of theory in HIV prevention. *AIDS Care*, **12**(3), 273–8.

Gillick v. West Norfolk and Wisbech Area Health Authority [1985] All ER 402.

Hancock, J. (2004) Can mainstream services learn from male only sexual health projects? *Sexually Transmitted Infections*, **80**, 484–7.

Hausser, D. and Michaud, P. (1994) Does a condom promoting strategy (the Swiss STOP-AIDS campaign) modify sexual behaviour among adolescents? *Paediatrics*, **93**(4), 580–5.

Health Protection Agency (2005) *Mapping the Issues: HIV and other Sexually Transmitted Infections in the UK: 2005*. http://www.hpa.org.uk/; accessed 24 August 2007.

Ingham, R., Clements, S. and Gillibrand, R. (2000) *Factors Affecting Changes in Rates of Teenage Conceptions 1991 to 1997*. Teenage Pregnancy Unit, London.

Kelly, E. (2001) The no-condom generation. *Cosmopolitan*, December, 136–42.

Kirby, D. (2001) *Emerging Answers: Research Findings on Programs to Reduce Unwanted Teenage Pregnancy*. National Campaign to Prevent Teen Pregnancy, Washington.

Lane, D. and and Day, P. (2001) Setting up a sexual health clinic in a school. *Nursing Times*, **97**(41), 38–9.

Lebrun-Vignes, B., Bouzamondo, A., Guillame, J., Lechat, P. Chosidow, O. (2007) A meta-analysis to assess the efficacy of oral antiviral treatment to prevent genital herpes outbreaks. *Journal of American Academy of Dermatology*, **57**(2), 238–44.

Lewis, D., McDonald, A., Thompson, G. and Bingham, J. (2004) The 374 clinic: an outreach sexual health clinic for young men. *Sexually Transmitted Infections*, **80**, 480–3.

Mahoney, C. (2000) Protection racket. *Nursing Times*, **96**(16), 30–1.

Mayor, S. (2004) Pregnancy and childbirth are leading causes of death in teenage girls in developing countries. *British Medical Journal*, **328**, 1152.

McCarney, E. and Hendee, W. (1989) Adolescent pregnancy and its consequences. *Journal of the American Medical Association*, **262**(1), 74–7.

Metcalfe, T. (2004) Sexual health: meeting adolescents' needs. *Nursing Standard,* **18**(46), 40–3.

Moens, V., Baruch, G. and Fearon, P. (2003) Opportunistic screening for chlamydia at a community based contraceptive service. *British Medical Journal,* **326**, 1252–5.

NICE (2007) *One to One Interventions to Reduce the Transmission of STIs Including HIV, and to Reduce the Rate of Under 18 Conceptions, Especially Among Vulnerable and At Risk Groups.* NICE Public Health Intervention Guidance 3, London.

Office for Standards in Education (2002) *Sex and Relationships.* HMI 433. Ofsted, London.

Paton, D. (2002) The economics of family planning and underage conceptions. *Journal of Health Economics,* **21**, 207–25.

Peckham, S., Ingham, R. and Diamond, I. (1996) *Teenage Pregnancy: Prevention and Programmes.* Institute for Health Policy Studies, University of Southampton.

Piaget, J. (1972) Intellectual evolution from adolescence to adulthood. *Human Development,* **15**(1), 1–12.

Rambout, L., Hopkins, L., Dutton, B. and Fergusson, D. (2007) Prophylactic vaccination against human papillomavirus infection and disease in women: a systematic review of randomized controlled trials. *CMAJ,* **177**(5), 469–79.

Sheffield Centre for HIV and Sexual Health (2007) Parent-to-Parent project. http://www.sexualhealthsheffield.nhs.uk/; accessed 31 August 2007.

Smith, A. (2006) Teenage girls call for compulsory sex education. *Guardian Unlimited,* Tuesday 28 February. http://www.education.guardian.co.uk/; accessed 24 May 2007.

Social Exclusion Unit (1999) *Teenage Pregnancy.* Home Office, London.

Stephenson, J., Imrie, J. and Bonell, C. (2003) *Effective Sexual Interventions: Issues in Experimental Evaluation.* Oxford University Press, Oxford.

Swann, C., Bowe, K., McCormick, G. and Kosmin, M. (2003) *Teenage Pregnancy and Parenthood: a Review of Reviews. Evidence Briefing.* Health Development Agency, London. http://www.hda.nhs.uk/; accessed 27 September 2007.

Stone, N. and Ingham, R. (2002) Factors affecting British teenagers' contraceptive use at first intercourse: the importance of partner communication. *Perspectives on Sexual and Reproductive Health,* **34**(4), 191–7.

Taylor, G. (2006) Sexual health is the message. *The Guardian,* Tuesday 30 May. http://www.education.guardian.co.uk/; accessed 6 September 2007.

Teenage Pregnancy Unit (2007) *Teenage Conception Statistics for England 1998–2005.* http://www.everychildmatters.gov.uk/; accessed 24 August 2007.

Thistle, S. and Ray, C. (2002) Sex and relationships education: the role of the school nurse. *Nursing Standard,* **17**(1), 44–53.

United Nation's Children's Fund (UNICEF) (2007) *A League Table of Teenage Births in Rich Nations.* Innocenti Report Card Three, Innocenti Research Centre, Florence.

University of York (1997) Preventing and reducing the adverse effects of unintended teenage pregnancy. *Effective Health Care,* **3**(1), 1–12.

Valk, G. (2000) *The Dutch Model.* Unesco the Courier. http://www.unesco.org/; accessed 24 May 2007.

van den Akker, O. B. A., Andre, J., Lees, S. and Murphy, T. (1999) Adolescent sexual behaviour and knowledge. *British Journal of Midwifery,* **7**(12), 765–9.

Wallmyr, G. and Welin, C. (2006) Young people, pornography and sexuality: sources and attitudes. *Journal of School Nursing*, **22**(5), 290–5.

Wellings, K., Field, J., Johnson, A. and Wadsworth, J. (1994) *Sexual Behaviour in Britain: the National Survey of Sexual Attitudes and Lifestyles.* Penguin, Harmondsworth.

Wellings, K., Nanchahal, K., Macdowall, W., McManus, S., Erens, R., Mercer, C., Johnson, A., Copas, A., Korovessis, C., Fenton, K. and Field, J. (2001) Sexual behaviour in Britain: early heterosexual experience. *Lancet*, (**358**), 1843–50.

White, J. (1987) Influence of parents, peers and problem solving on contraceptive use. *Paediatric Nursing*, **13**(5), 317–21.

Weyman, A. (2003) Promoting sexual health to young people: preventing teenage pregnancy and sexually transmitted infections. *Journal of the Royal Society for the Promotion of Health*, **123**(1), 6–11.

Whaley, L., Wong, D. and Hockenberry-Eaton, M. (1999) *Whaley and Wong's Nursing Care of Infants and Children*, 6th edn. Mosby, St Louis, MO.

Wright, S. (1999) Sexually transmitted diseases. *Nursing Standard*, **13**(46), 37–42.

CHAPTER 9

Child protection and the school-age child

Kate Potter

Key themes

- The historical context
- Definitions and concepts
- Physical abuse
- Emotional abuse
- Neglect
- Sexual abuse
- Domestic violence
- Working together for the best outcomes for children

Introduction

The guide to inter-agency working (HM Govt, 2006:11) clearly states:

> A shared responsibility and the need for effective joint working between agencies and professionals that have different roles and expertise are required if children are to be protected from harm and their welfare promoted.

During their years of formal education children come into contact with a variety of professionals from a number of agencies, both statutory and voluntary. Lord Laming (2003) underlined the need for greater accountability of all agencies in their role of protecting children from abuse. This requires all practitioners to have an understanding of both the procedures in the process of child protection and knowledge of underlying causes, risk factors and evidence of successful interventions. The aim of this chapter is to give an overview of this complex area and suggest further reading to expand practitioners' knowledge.

The historical context

The prevalence of child abuse has been a major concern throughout the developed world since the early 1960s (Lawrence, 2004) but there has been an awareness of the requirement for policy, legislation and structure to protect vulnerable children from a much earlier time. The industrialisation and urbanisation of Britain during the Victorian period resulted in increased poverty and a reduction in both community support and control (Corby, 2006). The informal welfare systems which existed to some extent within rural communities did not develop in the rapidly expanding cities and towns.

There was a growing awareness of cruelty to children among social reformers and philanthropists, but many felt that what occurred within the family should be regarded as private and thus beyond legislation. However, in 1883 Thomas Agnew set up the Liverpool Society for the Prevention of Cruelty to Children (NSPCC, 2007). The movement rapidly grew throughout the country. There then followed active campaigning and raising of public awareness about the lack of legislation to protect children within families and in 1889 the Prevention of Cruelty to Children Act was passed (Corby, 2006). Further Acts followed (see Table 9.1) and provided the framework for current child protection practice.

Lawrence (2004) refers to the current discourse in Child Protection arising from the aftermath of several child abuse cases in the 1970s and 1980s. The Maria Colwell case (Department of Health and Social Security, 1974) and the Jasmine Beckford inquiry report (Blom-Cooper, 1985) both had significant influence on child protection practice. The Cleveland affair resulted from the increasing awareness of both health and social work professionals of a much higher than previously thought incidence of sexual abuse. The inquiry, although warning of over-zealous practice, did recognise the importance of ensuring that protecting children from sexual abuse remained on the political agenda (Corby, 2006). The Laming Report (2003) is the most recent report and possibly had the highest media profile. Parton (2004) compares the reports and underlines that the key themes remain the confusion in working practice and the failure of professionals to communicate key information both within and across agencies. Significant recommendations for practitioners working with children have been incorporated into the latest Working Together Guide (HM Govt, 2006).

Table 9.1 The development of child protection.

1872	Infant Life Protection Act – to prevent Baby Farming
1883	Thomas Agnew founds the Liverpool Society for the Prevention of Cruelty to Children
1889	National Society for Prevention of Cruelty set up
1889	Children's Charter – State could arrest anyone found ill-treating a child
1894	Charter amended – Offence to deny child medical attention
1904	Prevention of Cruelty Act – NSPCC Inspectors granted permission to take children from abusive homes
1908	Children Act – Registration of Foster Parents. Sexual abuse within families to be dealt with by state
1933	Children Act – Supervision orders for children at risk
1948	Children Act Children's committee and Children's Officer in each local area
1962	Henry Kempe published work identifying 'the battered child syndrome'
1970	Social Services Act – Children's services amalgamated into social services departments
1974	Maria Colwell inquiry led to formation of Area Child Protection Committees
1985	Jasmine Beckwith Inquiry
1987	Kimberley Carlile and Tyra Henry inquiries
1988	Cleveland Inquiry
1989	Children Act – Rights of children. Focus on remaining with family
1999	Protection of Children Act – Aimed to prevent paedophiles working with children
2003	Laming Report – Leading to Green Paper: Every Child Matters
2004	The Children Act – To implement the proposals of the Green Paper
2005	Appointment of England's first children's commissioner

Children Act 1989 and Children Act 2004

The Children Act 1989 has provided the framework of legislation for the support and protection of children within the United Kingdom. It was a major change in direction as it attempted to balance the rights of children and parents and the need for a mechanism of state intervention when necessary (Lawrence, 2004). There is a great deal of focus on working with parents in an open manner and for the first time, parents would be included in case conferences. In addition to the consideration of parents' rights, the importance of children being given the opportunity to make choices and voice their feelings was emphasised.

The Children Act 2004 is viewed as a response from government to the repercussions following the death of Victoria Climbié (Brammer, 2007). The Act provides the legal underpinning for the policy set out in the Green Paper *Every Child Matters* (DfES, 2004). Shortly after this, the Every Child Matters website was launched, which provides support and guidance for the implementation of practice to achieve the five outcomes for all children. The 2004 Act focuses on ensuring good practice and integrated working across agencies. The establishment of the role of Children's Commissioner is a recognition that the views and interests of children are paramount for the five key outcomes of *Every Child Matters* to be achieved (Brammer, 2007).

Definitions and concepts

In *Working Together to Safeguard Children* (HM Govt, 2006, p. 34) it states that in all government legislation and guidelines a child is anyone who has not yet reached their 18th birthday. It should also be noted that in some instances the age is 21. This has implications for all professionals who work with young adults, including those within further education, prison services and the armed forces. The document focuses on Safeguarding and promoting the welfare of children and child protection.

This is seen as:

- Protecting children from maltreatment
- Preventing impairment of children's health and development
- Ensuring children are growing up in circumstances with the provision of safe and effective care.

Child protection is part of this process, but encompasses activities to protect children who are suffering, or at risk of suffering, significant harm. The document declines to provide absolute criteria for judging what constitutes significant harm but states that:

> Consideration of the severity of the ill-treatment may include the degree and the extent of the physical harm, the duration and frequency

of abuse and neglect, the extent of premeditation and the presence or degree of threat, coercion, sadism and bizarre and unusual elements (HM Govt, 2006, p. 36)

The child has to be the focus of the assessment and the effects of any behaviour by carers on their health and development will be vital to the judgements made. The four main categories of abuse are physical, sexual, emotional abuse and neglect.

Physical abuse

This may involve: hitting, shaking, throwing, poisoning, burning or scalding, drowning, suffocating, or otherwise causing physical harm to a child. Physical harm may also be caused when a parent fabricates the symptoms of, or deliberately induces illness in, a child (HM Govt, 2006, p. 37).

A quarter of children within the United Kingdom experience one or more forms of physical violence during their childhood (Cawson *et al.*, 2000). Although it has been acknowledged that children under one year are the most at risk from severe physical abuse, practitioners working with school-age children need to be aware that there is still a high incidence with children as they get older. However, as age increases, the chance of dying from Non Accidental Injury (NAI) decreases (Howe, 2005). In 2006 there were 5,100 children on the Child Protection Register under this category (DfES, 2004). The identification of NAI is not always straightforward. There is much debate as to what constitutes mild physical punishment, which was reflected in the consultation *Protecting Children, Supporting Parents* (DH, 2000). The guidance relates to context, severity, duration and age of the child. The wording in the document does not provide clarity to the extent that both parents and professionals may have considerable difficulty in determining what can be seen as acceptable chastisement (Cousins and Watkins, 2005).

Practitioners working in schools, primary health care settings or acute hospitals may be confronted with these decisions. Professionals need to be clear not only how to identify NAI but also how then to raise issues with both children and parents. Research has shown that within primary care this is an area of concern and often practitioners lack confidence in their own ability to diagnosis correctly (Russell *et al.*, 2004). Misdiagnosis can lead to failure to investigate properly, as in the case of Victoria Climbié (Laming, 2003), where sores and scars inflicted by her carers were erroneously attributed to scabies. It is important to be clear about what types of injury are most likely to have been inflicted deliberately, either as a result of over-zealous chastisement or for other more sinister reasons. The nature of the injury, its position on the body and the explanations given by the parent and child need all to be taken into account. Children may present with an injury which has obviously been sustained several days previously or have several bruises which have clearly been the result of trauma occurring at different times. Marks and scars may be observed by school staff or by nurses in accident and emergency units or in primary care, and it is important that if there are concerns they are followed up immediately. This can be problematic for school nurses who are not visiting schools on a daily basis. So all staff working within the education setting need to know how to respond appropriately.

Certain groups of children are at more risk from physical abuse. These include those with physical disabilities, learning disabilities, visual and hearing impairment, low birth weight, physical health problems and behavioural disorders, such as Attention Deficit Hyperactive Disorder (Howe, 2005). It is clear that caring for children in these categories is likely to be more stressful and it is often a result of inadequate support being given to the parents (National Working Group on Child Protection and Disability, 2003). Boys are more likely to be disciplined physically than girls (Watkins and Cousins, 2005). Children from lower socio-economic backgrounds were shown in a study by Cawson *et al.* (2000) to be more likely reported as being physically abused and neglected. It is arguable, however, that those living in more socially deprived areas are more open to state surveillance (Corby, 2006, p. 131).

Fabrication or induced illness, formerly often referred to as Munchausen by Proxy Syndrome, is also recognised as a form of physical abuse. This is a relatively rare form of abuse (Corby, 2006), but has a high profile because of the high risk of fatality to the child involved. The abuse is likely to start when the children are very young and 77% of identified cases are noted before the age of five years (DH, 2002), but there will be incidences which are not detected until the child reaches school age. Carers who abuse children in this way have often been abused themselves and may also have a history of psychiatric illness, often somatising and personality disorder (Howe, 2005).

The Department of Health (2002, p. 13) gives the following list of behaviours that are part of this type of abuse:

- Deliberately inducing symptoms in children by administering medication or other substances, or by means of intentional suffocation.
- Interfering with treatment by over dosing, not administering them or interfering with medical equipment such as infusion lines.
- Claiming the child has symptoms which are unverifiable unless observed directly, such as pain, frequency of passing urine vomiting or fits. These claims result in unnecessary investigations and treatments, which may cause secondary physical problems.
- Exaggerating symptoms, causing professionals to undertake investigations and treatments, which may be invasive, are unnecessary and therefore are harmful and possibly dangerous.

- Obtaining specialist treatment or equipment for children who do not require them.
- Alleging psychological illness in the child.

It is important to remember that fabrication or induction of illness can be by a carer such as a foster parent or child minder, or a nurse, as in the case of Beverley Allitt, who murdered four children and injured many more on a paediatric ward in England in the early 1990s (Ferner, 2002). Although this is a rare occurrence in children over five, it is important, especially for health professionals working in the acute sector, to be aware of the significance of frequently reported, but not seen symptoms. Older children may also develop abnormal attitudes to their own health (Howe, 2005).

Emotional abuse

The definition of emotional abuse is clear and comprehensive (HM Govt, 2006, p. 38):

> the persistent emotional maltreatment of a child such as to cause severe and persistent adverse effects on the child's emotional development. It may involve conveying to children that they are worthless or unloved, inadequate or valued only insofar as they meet the needs of another person. It may feature age or developmentally inappropriate expectations being imposed on children. These may include interactions that are beyond the child's developmental capability, as well as overprotection and limitation of exploration and learning, or preventing the child participating in normal social interaction. It may involve the seeing or hearing of mistreatment of another. It may involve serious bullying, causing children frequently to feel frightened or in danger, or the exploitation or corruption of children. Some level of emotional abuse is involved in all types of maltreatment of a child, though it may occur alone.

This definition clearly underlines the harm which can be caused by domestic violence, which will be explored later in this chapter, and also by expectations of children taking on a caring role beyond their capabilities. School nurses and other professionals working in education are often the first to be aware that a child is looking after a younger sibling or a parent with mental health problems. It is acknowledged that professionals have difficulty in clearly articulating concerns to ensure adequate intervention where they fear that a child is being emotionally abused (Corby, 2006). Griffin and Tyrrell (2002) offer the

Human Givens Approach which suggests that the basic emotional needs for all human beings are:

- Security and safety
- Attention
- Connection with others
- A sense of belonging and status
- Being psychologically stretched
- A balance between autonomy and control
- A sense of purpose and meaning – usually based in good relationships

These 'human givens' provide a focus for practitioners who need to clearly identify what their concerns are when they feel a child may be suffering from emotional abuse.

The effects of long-term emotional abuse are far reaching and are intrinsically linked with attachment and the development of the emotional brain, which are outlined in another chapter of this book. Children who have been emotionally abused will struggle with peer relationships and it is likely that this may continue, if there are no interventions, into adult life, which may subsequently affect their relationship with their own children (Howe, 2005). O'Hagan (2006, p. 48) debates that emotionally abused children are likely to function at 'either extreme of an emotional spectrum'. She describes those who have 'silent and invisible' negative emotions and whose negative emotions are 'audible and visible'. The former appear to those who work with them as withdrawn and emotionless, as they have learned that displaying emotion will elicit a negative response from abusive carers, within the school setting, these children may well not be identified as needing help. Children who display their negative emotions audibly and for all to see by being uncontrollable and aggressive are much more likely to be noticed and hopefully receive appropriate support and interventions. It is clear then, that anyone who works with children, needs to understand what constitutes normal emotional behaviour and be aware of all children whose emotional responses may be due to abusive relationships. These children need to be assessed and referred to the appropriate level of Child and Mental Health services.

Neglect

This is the most common category of child abuse. Children who were the subject of a child protection plan in England because of neglect totalled 11,800 out of 26,400 in 2006 (NSPCC, 2007a). Neglect is defined as:

The persistent failure to meet a child's basic physical and/or psychological needs, likely to result in the serious impairment of the child's health or development (HM Govt, 2006, p. 38).

Neglect may occur during pregnancy as a result of maternal substance abuse. Once a child is born, neglect may involve a parent or carer failing to:

- Provide adequate food clothing and shelter (including exclusion from home or abandonment)
- Protect a child from physical and emotional harm and danger
- Ensure adequate supervision (including the use of inadequate care givers)
- Ensure access to appropriate medical care or treatment.

It may also include neglect of or unresponsiveness to a child's basic emotional needs.

The interpretation of this definition can vary amongst professionals and the threshold of what is acceptable can prove contentious (Howarth, 2005). This is confirmed by research that shows that practitioners do not agree on which particular circumstances would constitute the need for referral (Stone, 1998). In the research, it was found that there was no one factor of neglect which could be taken on its own as being significant enough to warrant referral. Stone (1998, p. 49) came to the conclusion that:

Neglect may therefore be considered to be a loosely defined category indicative of professional concern about standard of childcare. This indicates that adequate clinical supervision for practitioners is vital in order that support can be given on what constitutes adequate parenting.

If we return to the inter-agency guidelines definition (HM Govt, 2006) it is clear that neglect is likely to be something that carries on over a period of time. Neglect has to be assessed from an understanding of child development, both physically and emotionally. A five-year-old child should not be expected to get their own breakfast and make their way to school, but this could be acceptable for a fourteen year old. In secondary schools, lack of control and boundaries for adolescents become concerns for practitioners and often parents. Parenting classes provided within the education setting allow parents to gain skills and confidence in appropriately supporting their children and also providing them with secure boundaries. Teenagers who are pregnant may require extra support to understand the needs both of themselves and of their unborn child. They are less likely to engage with antenatal services and may have less support in the postnatal period.

It has been recognised that there are certain factors that increase the risk of parents becoming neglectful of their children. Crittenden (1999) divides neglect into three types: families who are disorganised, those who are depressed and those who are emotionally neglectful. Families who fall into the category of being neglectful because they are disorganised are the most likely to already have had input from a variety of services. They have chaotic lifestyles and it is this chaos which often results in the needs of the child, whether physical or emotional, not being met (Stevenson, 2007). Crittenden's category of depressed neglect is not specifically related to particular mental health problems, but is more to do with an overall attitude which does not allow for any decision making to take control of their own lives. These parents and carers find it difficult to attend medical appointments or ensure that their children arrive at school on time, and are unlikely without support to engage in any activities within the school setting. The practitioner may feel sympathy towards the parent and be reluctant to make referrals, but the needs of the child must be paramount.

Although it is not always the case, there is an increased risk that parents with mental health problems and those who abuse drugs and alcohol will neglect their children both physically and emotionally (Howe, 2005). It is important to consider what factors are likely to increase the risk, this will include looking at social support networks, whether the family is in stable accommodation and in the case of drug and alcohol abuse exposure to other users (Stevenson, 2007). Close working between children's workers and members of mental health teams can help to ensure that proper risk assessments are made. Again, it is important to have an empathetic approach to the problems of the parents, but always in the context of both the short- and long-term consequences for the children.

A key issue for practitioners arises around parents who have learning disabilities. They are more likely to have their children taken into care than any other parents (Macdonald, 2005). Concerns are often raised around the ability they have to meet their children's physical and emotional needs and protect them from harm (Stevenson, 2007). Practitioners need to be aware of the difficulties which these parents face and provide adequate support. The adolescent child may become increasingly challenging and extra support in parenting skills may be required. Children who have disabilities themselves are statistically more likely to suffer from neglect (Sullivan and Nutson, 1998). This is often due to the lack of support which their carers are given with the cost to the family both physically and emotionally not always being recognised. Practitioners who work with children with disabilities need to be aware of all the services, both statutory and voluntary, available to provide adequate support for families. They have a key role in responsibly carrying out a full assessment and ensuring that all available services are provided for the family. This includes helping parents contact carers' support groups and specific organisations for particular physical and mental conditions. Parents of disabled children frequently feel isolated, and contact with other parents in similar conditions can not only provide practical support but also alleviate these feelings of being socially isolated. This is explored further in Chapter 10.

Sexual abuse

In 2006 there were 2,600 registrations to child protection registers under the category of sexual abuse (NSPCC, 2007a). This is the smallest number of any of the abuse categories, but it is widely believed that there is a much more widespread problem in which abuse of a sexual nature often remains undetected (Lawrence, 2004). Cawson *et al.* (2000) found that 1% of children under 16 experience abuse. There is a much higher rate for girls than boys (21% as opposed to 11%) and the majority of children from both sexes who have been abused will have been so on more than one occasion. In this research it was found that the rate of disclosure was low, with only 28% reporting the abuse at the time and 31% still not sharing their experience when they were adults. In 2006 the NSPCC launched the 'Don't hide it' website. The results of a survey carried out on this website indicated that sex education in schools did not fully address sexual abuse, leaving children confused and less likely to report inappropriate incidents (NSPCC, 2006).

According to the inter-agency guidance (HM Govt, 2006, p. 38):

Sexual abuse involves forcing or enticing a child or young person to take part in sexual activities, including prostitution, whether or not the child is aware of what is happening. The activities may involve physical contact, including penetrative (e.g. rape, buggery or oral sex) or non-penetrative acts. They may include non-contact activities, such as involving children in looking at, or in the production of sexual on-line images, watching sexual activities, or encouraging children to behave in sexually inappropriate ways.

Research shows that the most likely perpetrators will be known to the child. This may be a family member often a brother, father, stepbrother or step father.

Unless a child discloses sexual abuse there are few clear signs to alert practitioners (Corby, 2006). Practitioners are often alerted by what is considered to be inappropriate sexual behaviour, but with older children there is more debate on what is considered to be inappropriate (Corby, 2006). The NSPCC (2005) provide useful guidelines on what constitutes normal sexual behaviour in different age groups and also suggests what may cause concern, including sexually explicit language in children younger than six and adult-like sexual behaviour in pre-adolescent children. The reporting of frequent urinary tract infections in girls and enuresis in both sexes may alert health practitioners, but it is important to exclude all other causes before raising suspicion.

Disclosure of sexual abuse is likely to happen when a trusting relation-ship has been built between a child and an adult. School nurses, children's nurses and practitioners working within CAMHS may find that they are the first person that a child has been able to disclose the abuse to. It is impor-tant that all professionals working with children are adequately trained so that they know that the correct procedures are adhered to, both to ensure the least trauma to the child and so that evidence for future prosecution is collected appropriately (HM Govt 2006) Children need to be listened to with respect and clear and comprehensive records kept. They need to be informed that a referral needs to be made and the process needs to be explained. If a child does require medical examination this needs to be undertaken as soon as possible by an appropriately qualified paediatrician to ensure that the examination only has to be carried out on one occasion. Parents or carers may also disclose concerns and it is important to be aware of whether any other children are at risk.

The increase in child prostitution and child trafficking is causing concern for all professionals who work with children (UNICEF, 2004). Reports in 2007 show that the problem is increasing and often vulnerable adolescents become lost to the system. The guide to inter-agency working (HM Govt, 2006, p. 148) underlines that these children must be treated as victims of abuse and those who are involved in their exploitation must be prosecuted. Children may have arrived in the country accompanied by adults known to their families, but they are often frightened of their traffickers and exploiters and so are reluctant to give any information. Practitioners may become aware of a child who is in the care of someone who is not a relative or by an adult who is controlling their movements and inappropriately influencing their behaviour. These children may well not attend school and may only come into contact with profession-als when unwell. The NSPCC provides an advice and information line, which provides guidance for anyone who has concerns.

The Sex Offences Act 2003 was passed to help protect children from abus-ers who use internet chat rooms to groom their victims. All children and par-ents need to be aware of the dangers. The internet can now be accessed not only from home computers but also mobile phones. This means that parents have less knowledge of what sites are being used and content filters are unavailable for all technology. One in five children between the ages of 9 and 16 regularly use internet chat rooms, and of these one in ten is likely to arrange a face-to-face meeting with another user. There is also increasing concern about ready access to pornographic material (Dombrowski *et al.*, 2007). School settings are the obvious setting for providing education and guidance in all aspects of the safe use of the internet. The NSPCC also provides a Safe Surfing Guide aimed at both parents and children.

Domestic violence

Over the last twenty years there has been an increasing amount of research carried out on the effect of domestic violence on children (Radford and Hester, 2006). Despite an increasing awareness of the problem, two women a week are killed by a current or former partner, 52% of all child protection cases involve domestic violence and in 90% of domestic violence incidents the children are in the same or an adjacent room (DH, 2005). It is also important to recognise the link between domestic violence and physical abuse for children. Some studies have put the link at a rate between 30% and 66% (Women's Aid, 2005). The impact of domestic violence on children varies depending on their age and stage of development (Humphreys and Stanley, 2006). There is also a difference in the ways that boys and girls react when experiencing living with domestic violence. Boys are more likely to become aggressive and disobedient and may also attempt to use violence to solve problems. As they reach adolescence they are also likely to truant and abuse drugs and alcohol. Girls have a tendency to internalise their feelings and become anxious and depressed. They are likely to have low self-esteem and be at a greater risk than normal of developing eating disorders or adopting self-harming behaviour. Both sexes are likely to do less well than their peers at school (Royal College of Psychiatrists, 2004).

There is much debate as to whether children raised in families where there is domestic violence get drawn into a cycle of abuse (Radford and Hester, 2006). Research has indicated that men who are violent in relationships are more likely to have been exposed to violence in childhood (Humphreys and Stanley, 2006). Although it is recognised that this should not be regarded as a definite cause of domestic violence, it has been acknowledged that there is an important role for those who work with school children in preventative work. The recommendations from the document *Tackling Domestic Violence; Effective Interventions and Approaches* (Hester and Westmarland, 2005) are that work with children on healthy relationships should be carried out at both primary and secondary school levels. The document describes projects which have not only raised awareness of domestic violence issues but have also, often through drama groups, provided skills in non-violent conflict resolution and challenged sexist attitudes. Research has shown that many adolescent boys condone violence in relationships, and often this is also accepted by girls (Mullender *et al.*, 2002). The recommendations of the report are that primary prevention of domestic violence, which includes addressing these attitudes, should not only be included in the PSHE curriculum but also with a much broader perspective, taking a cross-curricular approach. There is a specific role for school nurses and other practitioners with a particular expertise in domestic violence awareness training in developing these strategies within schools. Children who are witnessing domestic violence at home need to be given the opportunity to talk and raise their concerns (Mullender, 2004). They often find support from schools variable and some children do not feel listened to (Humphreys and Stanley, 2006). They often feel isolated from their classmates and avoid making close relationships with other children as they feel the need to keep their family situation secret (Buckley *et al.*, 2007). Drop-in clinics where children feel safe to disclose their concerns can be invaluable. Children may want to address the ambivalent feelings which they have towards the perpetrator of the violence and the emotional confusion which they are experiencing. (Radford and Hester, 2006). A significant amount of work is done by Women's Aid, both within refuge settings and as outreach work in this area. They have also created 'Hide Out': a web-based resource which can be accessed by children. The practitioner should be aware of these resources and make them generally available in the school setting. Children who are living in refuges and attending local schools will also often need extra support as they will be isolated from their extended family and friends and will need to adjust to a new school environment.

Working together for the best outcomes for children

The report on the death of Victoria Climbié (Laming, 2003) underlined the need for professionals to communicate with appropriate agencies when there were concerns regarding the welfare of a child. The response to this has been to place more emphasis on training and development for inter- and multi-agency working (HM Govt, 2006). Guidance in the *Working Together* document underlines that all staff working directly with children, including hospital and community health staff, teachers and mental health and learning disability staff should have:

> A higher minimum level of expertise: a fuller understanding of how to work together to identify and assess concerns and to plan, undertake and review interventions (HM Govt, 2006, p. 95).

Practitioners need therefore to ensure that they undertake the offered training, which should ensure that they are fully aware of their roles and responsibilities. They should be supported by their own area guidelines of practice and have access to a named specialist who can be contacted for advice at any time. The role of Local Safeguarding Children's Boards to ensure that this framework is in place is clear (HM Govt, 2006). The Common Assessment Framework (CWDC, 2007) should be used for assessing the needs of children when concerns for their safety are not immediate and also may help to identify concerns when making a referral if there are child protection issues.

Inter-agency and multi-disciplinary conflict often arises around referrals (Lawrence, 2004). Concerns need to be clearly articulated and this is often dependent on accurate and contemporaneous record keeping. Referrals need to be tracked and they need to be owned by the person who has concerns. It is vital that all relevant information communicated, including telephone call and face-to-face conversations should be recorded with accuracy (Newland, 2007). School nurses and health visitors are often viewed by other health professionals as having more expertise in the area of child protection, and this is often the case, but they should provide support for teachers or voluntary workers to make the referrals themselves. If a case conference is called practitioners should provide an accurate report, written with adherence to local guidelines and with the support of the named nurse for child protection. The contents of the report should be shared with the parents prior to the conference. If the case conference decides that the child should be the subject of a protection plan, it is likely that the health practitioner will be part of the core group and will have the opportunity to work with the family and other agencies to achieve the best outcomes for the child.

Conclusion

The need to safeguard children from harm has been recognised for almost 200 years. The development of a framework for child protection has often been a response to inquiries following deaths of children as a result of the failure of systems in place at the time. Over the last thirty years there has been a growing body of research into the causes of abuse and which interventions are most effective to produce best long-term outcomes for abused children. There is also an increased emphasis on prevention of abuse by addressing social exclusion and improving early childhood support. Practitioners have a role within school settings to discuss healthy relationships with children of all ages and prepare them for a future role as parents. Along with this, it is important to listen to children, observe their behaviour and assess whether they may be in a situation which could cause them significant harm.

References

Brammer, A. (2007) *Social Work Law*, 2nd edn. Pearson Education, Harlow.
Blom-Cooper, L. (1985) *A Child in Trust*. Brent, London.

Buckley, H., Holt, S. and Whelan, S. (2007) Listen to me! Children's experiences of domestic violence. *Child Abuse Review*. **16**, 296–310.

Cawson, P., Wattam, C., Brooker, S. and Kelly, G. (2000) *Child Maltreatment in the United Kingdom: a Study of the Prevalence of Child Abuse and Neglect*. NSPCC, London.

Children's Workforce Development Council (2007) *Common Assessment Framework for Children and Young People: Practitioners' Guide*. CWDC, London.

Corby, B. (2006)*Child Abuse: Towards a Knowledge Base*. Open University Press, Maidenhead.

Cousins, J. and Watkins, D. (2005) Macrotheories: child physical punishment, injury and abuse. *Community Practitioner*. **78**(8), 276–9.

Crittenden, P. (1999) Child neglect: causes and contributors. In: *Neglected Children, Research, Practice and Policy* (ed. H. Dubowitz). Sage, California.

Department of Health/Department for Education and Skills (2004) *Every Child Matters*. DfES, London.

Department of Health (2000) *Protecting Children, Supporting Parents: a Consultation Document on the Physical Punishment of Children*. Department of Health, London.

Department of Health (2002) *Safeguarding Children in Whom Illness is Fabricated or Induced*. Department of Health, London.

Department of Health (2005) *Responding to Domestic Abuse. A Handbook for Professionals*. Department of Health, London.

Department of Health and Social Security (1975) *Report of the Committee of Inquiry into the Care and Supervision Provided in Relation to Maria Colwell*. HMSO, London.

Department for Education and Skills (2006) *Statistics of Education: Referrals, Assessment and Children and Young People on Child Protection Registers. Year Ending 31st March 2006*. DfES, London.

Dombrowski, S., Gischlar, K. and Durst, T. (2007) Safeguarding young people from cyber pornography and cyber sexual predation: a major dilemma of the internet. *Child Abuse Review*, **16**, 153–70.

Ferner, R. (2001) Our poisoned patients. *QJM: An International Journal of Medicine*. **94**, 117–20.

Griffin, J. and Tyrrell, L. (2002) *Psychotherapy and the Human Givens*, 2nd edn. HG Publishing, Chalvington.

HM Government (2006) *Working Together to Safeguard Children: A Guide to Interagency Working to Safeguard and Promote the Welfare of Children*. Stationery Office, London.

Hester, M. and Westmarland, N. (2005) *Tackling Domestic Violence: Effective Interventions and Approaches. Home Office Research Study 290*. Home Office, London.

Howe, D. (2005) *Child Abuse and Neglect: Attachment, Development and Intervention*. Palgrave Macmillan, London.

Howarth, J. (2005) Is this child neglect? The influence of differences in perception of child neglect on social work practice. In: *Child Neglect: Practice Issues for Health and Social Care* (eds. J. Taylor and B. Daniel). Jessica Kingsley, London.

Humphreys, C. and Stanley, N. (2006) *Domestic Violence and Child Protection. Directions for Good Practice*. Jessica Kingsley, London.

Laming, Lord (2003) *The Victoria Climbié Inquiry: Report of an Inquiry by Lord Laming.* Stationery Office, London.

Lawrence, A. (2004) *Principles of Child Protection. Management and Practice.* Open University Press, Maidenhead.

Macdonald, G. (2005) Intervening with neglect. In: *Child Neglect: Practice Issues for Health and Social Care* (eds. J. Taylor and B. Daniel). Jessica Kingsley, London.

Minty, B. (2005) The nature of emotional child neglect and abuse. In: *Child Neglect: Practice Issues for Health and Social Care* (eds. J. Taylor and B. Daniel). Jessica Kingsley, London.

Mullender, A., Hague, G., Iman, U., Kelly, L., Malos, E. and Regan, L. (2002) *Children's Perspectives on Domestic Violence.* Sage, London.

National Society for the Prevention of Cruelty to Children (2005) *Protecting Children from Sexual Abuse.* NSPCC, London.

NSPCC (2006) *Schools Fail to Teach Children About Sexual Abuse Finds NSPCC.* http://www.nspcc.org.uk/whatwedo/mediacentre/pressreleases/05_june_2006_schools_fail_to_teach_children_about_sexual_abuse_finds_nspcc_wdn33564.htm; accessed 29 December 2007.

National Society for the Prevention of Cruelty to Children (2007) *A Pocket History of the NSPCC.* http://www.nspcc.org.uk/; accessed 27 November 2007.

National Society for the Prevention of Cruelty to Children (2007a) *Child Protection Register Statistics – England 2003–2007.* NSPCC, London.

National Working Group on Child Protection and Disability (2003) *'It Doesn't Happen to Disabled Children'. Child Protection and Disabled Children.* NSPCC, London.

Newland, R. (2007) *Record Keeping and Documentation: Principles into Practice.* CPHVA, London.

O'Hagan K (2006) *Identifying Emotional and Psychological Abuse.* Open University Press, Maidenhead.

Parton, N. (2004) From Maria Colwell to Victoria Climbié: reflections on a generation of public inquiries into child abuse. *Child Abuse Review*, **13**(2), 80–94.

Radford, L. and Hester, M. (2006) *Mothering Through Domestic Violence.* Jessica Kingsley, London.

Royal College of Psychiatrists (2004) *Domestic Violence: Its Effects on Children. Factsheet for Parents and Teachers.* Royal College of Psychiatry, London.

Russell, M., Lazenbatt, A., Freeman, R. and Marcenes, W. (2004) Child physical abuse: health professionals' perceptions, diagnosis and responses. *British Journal of Community nursing*, **9**(8), 32–8.

Stevenson, O. (2007) *Neglected Children and Their Families.* Blackwell, London.

Stone, B. (1998) *Child Neglect: Practitioners' Perspectives.* NSPCC, London.

Sullivan, P. and Nutson, J. (1998)The association between child maltreatment and disabilities in a hospital based epidemiological study. *Child Abuse and Neglect*, **22**, 271–88.

UNICEF (2004) *The State of the World's Children 2005 – Childhood Under Threat.* UNICEF.

Women's Aid (2005) *Domestic Violence. Frequently Asked Questions. Fact Sheet.* Women's Aid, London.

Useful websites

Carers UK: http://www.carersuk.org/
Connexions Direct: http://www.connexions-direct.com/
Every Child Matters. Change for Children: http://www.everychildmatters.gov.uk/
General Social Care Council: http://www.gscc.org.uk/
Home Office: http://www.homeoffice.gov.uk/
The Hideout: http://www.thehideout.org.uk/
National Society for the Prevention of Cruelty to Children: http://www.nspcc.org.uk/
Joseph Rowntree Foundation: http://www.jrf.org.uk/
Parenting UK: http://www.parentinguk.org/
Women's Aid: http://www.womensaid.org.uk/

CHAPTER 10

Supporting the child with complex needs

Jane Wright and Liz Numadi

Key themes

- Supporting school-aged children with complex health and social needs in the community
- Barriers to achieving optimum health
- Perceptions of health
- Working together

Introduction

The aim of this chapter is to explore the concept of promoting the health of school-age children with complex needs, together with their families. Although defining complex needs is difficult, for the purposes of this chapter they are defined as problems which are likely to affect health, well-being, developmental milestones, social interactions and educational attainment. This includes children with special medical, educational and social needs, which may require additional support from different agencies. As the topic is so broad, a table is included as a resource in terms of treatment and support networks for groups of conditions (see Table 10.1). The intention of this chapter is to provide an overview and guide the reader to further resources and information.

It has been recognised that it is difficult to determine accurately the number of children requiring long-term health or social care at a specific point in time (Department of Health [DH], 2000; Hewitt-Tayor, 2005). However, the Department for Work and Pensions estimated that in 2003–2004 there were 700,000 children with disabilities and complex medical and social needs (Department for Work Pensions [DWP], 2006). It is also acknowledged that many chil-

Table 10.1 Children with complex needs.

Nature of complex need	Examples of diseases/ conditions	Likely duration	Symptoms
Lifelong chronic illness from birth	Congenital malformations (may resolve through surgical correction before adulthood) Cystic fibrosis Haemophilia Sickle cell anaemia Liver, gut or renal failure requiring intervention or transplant Cerebral palsy	Lifelong	Varying between daily control of symptoms required to remission/ relapse presentation to acute on chronic presentation
Long-term chronic illness from childhood	Inflammatory bowel disease Diabetes	May present from pre-school but more usually from later school age and pre-puberty for life	Relapse/remission pattern of symptoms
Chronic illness potentially limited to childhood	Asthma Eczema	May present as infantile symptoms or may continue into preschool age group with less children significantly affected beyond early school age	Generally acute on chronic presentation but may be severe with lifestyle limiting impact
Acute presentation with potential long term implications for care	Prematurity Epilepsy Correctable cardiac disorders Trauma/accidents requiring rehabilitation	Initial high intervention with serious consequences for lifestyle resolving to require long-term follow up	Following identification and adherence to treatment regime limitation on lifestyle may remain evident following rehabilitation
Malignant disease and life-threatening/ limiting illness	Leukaemia Muscular dystrophy HIV Inborn errors of metabolism	Strict regimes of management limiting life choices required to control/delay progression of disease	Acute illness which may be limited with treatment and may resolve or settles into pattern of long term progressive deterioration of function
Behavioural and emotional disorders	Attention deficit disorder Anorexia nervosa Autism	May be lifelong with varying impact during different times of life, e.g. puberty	Insidious onset with often delayed diagnosis with periods of deterioration associated with stimuli specific to child
Technology-dependent	Short gut requiring parenteral nutrition Congenital syndromes requiring ventilatory support Severe neurological injury requiring ventilation and nutritional intervention	Likely to be lifelong	Varying dependent on primary disorder, but all requiring high-tech intervention at home with specialist support

Nursing care	Social implications	Educational requirements	Referral required
Periods of high intervention required during acute illness Key role in coordination of services and support	May limit usual childhood activities limiting access to play and making friends Will be 'different' Possible pubertal growth delay	Varying need: perhaps School nurse LEA statement Hospital school Home tutor	Paediatrician or specialist paediatric consultant School nurse Dietician Physiotherapist Specialist children's nurse
Limited to acute episodes of relapse but essential to advocate with other agencies to meet requirements	May limit usual childhood activities limiting access to play and making friends Will be 'different' Possible pubertal growth delay	Varying need: perhaps School nurse Hospital school Home tutor	Paediatrician or specialist paediatric consultant School nurse Dietician Specialist children's nurse if available
Health promotion activities to limit exacerbation of condition Health education to empower families	May limit usual childhood activities limiting access to play and making friends	School nurse Maybe hospital school	Paediatrician School nurse Specialist childrens nurse
High level of intervention during critical illness/ stabilisation then ongoing support if requested	May severely limit usual childhood activities limiting access to play and making friends for some duration and may require major readjustment to lifestyle	Liaison with school nurse for awareness of specific need, e.g. mobility, administration of medication	Paediatrician or specialist paediatric consultant School nurse Dietician Physiotherapist Specialist children's nurse
High level of intervention and coordination during initial diagnosis and establishing plan of care and likely to continue during periods of deterioration	May limit usual childhood activities limiting access to play and making friends Family interaction may always be affected by fear of deterioration or death	School nurse for reintegration within school as needs change	Paediatrician or specialist paediatric consultant School nurse Dietician Physiotherapist Specialist children's nurse/Macmillan
Often specialist services provided although healthcare support can be limited in many areas	May severely limit usual childhood activities limiting access to play and making friends Huge emotional demand on all members of family	Varying need: perhaps School nurse LEA statement Residential care/ schooling	Paediatrician or specialist paediatric consultant School nurse CAMHS Specialist nurse
Usually provided by agency or company employed nurses can have impact on continuity of care	May severely limit ability to leave the house usually intervention is timed to occur predominately at night where feasible	Home tuition may be only option although school attendance likely if intermittent intervention only each day required	Specialist paediatric consultant Dietician Physiotherapist Specialist children's nurse

dren with complex needs have changed long-term health outcomes which include extended life expectancies into adolescence and adulthood (Valentine and Lowes, 2007). For example, the life expectancy for children with cystic fibrosis thirty years ago was six years, while in 2007 it was thirty-two years (Harrop, 2007). This will be a new field of experience for health and social care practitioners requiring further research and resources and it will continue to increase the demand for health and social care services and add financial pressure on the NHS (Wanless, 2002, 2007).

Improving care pathways and creating more effective community-based services are crucial to the ongoing care of children with complex needs to improve re-admission rates and improve quality of life (Chandler, 2007). Since the Wanless report in 2002, there has been a shift in policy towards more patient choice and self-care and a decentralisation of funding. This is in line with more cost-effective care using marketing principles with a maintained emphasis on quality and governance. Changes to community services, for example, include the introduction of Practice Based Commissioning (DH, 2004, 2005a). This is a process by which, it is suggested, organisations can identify the specific health needs of their population in order to make prioritised decisions regarding resources to meet need. In theory, this is an important development in the care of children and young people with ongoing complex needs and will help to develop more innovative models of care (DH, 2006a). Alongside practice-based commissioning, *Modernising Nursing Careers* (DH, 2006b) reviewed the education and development of nursing into the future. This also includes considering improvements in the care of people with complex needs, emphasising health promotion and supporting self-care using more flexible ways of working. The National Institute for Clinical Health Excellence (NICE) also influences the standards of care for children with complex health needs. For example producing guidelines on the care of children with cancer, eating disorders, diabetes, epilepsy and atopic eczema (NICE, 2008). Working in partnership is vital for promoting the health and well-being of children and families and is implicit within the *National Service Framework for Children, young people and Maternity Services*, standard 8, which states:

> Children and young people who are disabled or who have complex health needs should receive co-ordinated , high quality child and family centred services which are based on assessed needs, which promote social inclusion and where possible enable them and their families to live ordinary lives as close to home as possible (DH/DfES, 2004a, p. 7).

However, the evidence so far has been that standards in care across the country have varied and there is a long way to go before the required standards of care are met nationally (Davidson, 2003; Hall and Elliman, 2006; Wanless,

2007; Debell, 2007). This chapter is an overview of the support that children and young people with complex needs require. The concepts of health promotion will be discussed in relation to this and some recommendations for working practices in health and social care will be explored.

Figure 10.1 is a summary of the overall concepts relating to promoting the health of school aged children with complex needs and the factors which will affect this.

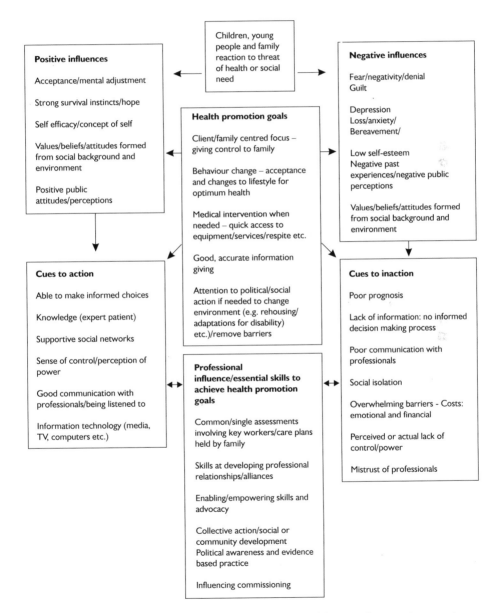

Figure 10.1 Promoting the health of school-age children with complex needs.

Promoting health

Promoting and improving the health and well-being of individuals and their families has been part of the public health agenda for decades and is both implicit and explicit throughout government health and social care strategies (DH, 2001; DH/DfES, 2004b; DH, 2006a). Traditional health promotion actions cannot be confined to parts of the population that are considered 'well', but must be inclusive of the whole population and therefore, have to be considered within a context of illness as well as health. The notion that there is a continuum between 'well' and 'diseased' and that the concept of being healthy is an entirely subjective one was described by Antonovsky (1984) (Cited in Sidell *et al.*, 2003) as the salutogenic paradigm. He was discussing the idea that the elderly are often labelled as unhealthy simply because they reported having a disability or long-term health problem. In reality, many of these people felt healthy, and this reinforces the concept of health as not simply the absence of disease but encompassing ideas of well-being and contentment. The salutogenic approach examines why, given similar circumstances, people will react differently to their situations or health conditions. This means a consideration of what being healthy means to individuals and how people adapt to their environment and construct meaningful lives around their difficulties (see Figure 10.1). Some parents of young people with complex health needs for example, may identify positive aspects of the experience, drawing on family strengths and adopting healthier lifestyles for themselves (Valentine and Lowes, 2007). Others may lack the coping strategies to deal with these difficulties, become ill themselves with stress-related conditions or feel that they have lost their identity as they struggle to cope (Hodgkinson and Lester, 2002). This may be related to barriers, either actual or perceived, by individuals and their families.

The concepts of family and child-centred care have moved towards combining social, medical and educational models where care is no longer 'done to or for' but 'done with' clients. This has been an attempt to move away from a bio-medical model of health where conditions are treated out of the context of individual circumstances. This has also been described as developing shared responsibility or authority where professional and personal boundaries are negotiated with the clear aim of improving the health outcomes for individuals and their families (Peate and Whiting, 2006). Each case needs to be examined and negotiated on its own merit and assumptions should not be made that all families are willing or able to cope alone, but that partnerships are developed to provide quality care (Hall and Elliman, 2006). This includes consideration of many factors such as cultural background, social circumstances and available support networks, including professional, family or voluntary.

Families have reported difficulties with support and respite care (DWP, 2007) which, in turn, leads to more returns to hospital, and potentially poor attention to the developmental and educational needs of children and young people. The barriers may be related to a range of problems, such as difficulty accessing information, language and cultural differences, belonging to a disadvantaged group such as black and ethnic minorities or those living in poverty (Joseph Rowntree Foundation [JRF], 2002; Davidson, 2003; DH, 2007b).

There also needs to be consideration of the most appropriate person to support families, not only those best qualified to support individual family circumstances within a multi-agency team, but also who the family is most likely to respond to (Carter *et al.*, 2007). This may mean a shift in thinking, particularly for professionals unwilling to relinquish their control. Recognising differences in the way people both perceive and cope with their situation is a vital component of family-centred care and is a concept explored on both pre-registration nursing and social care courses.

A more coordinated approach to assessing individual need has come in the form of the Common Assessment Framework (CAF). This has arisen out of the *Framework for Assessing Children in Need and their Families* (DH, 2000) document. It is an attempt to promote a more effective identification of specific needs for children and families; in particular, to be able to identify the services required to meet these needs by negotiating with children and parents and listening to what is important for them. This assessment tool was formally piloted during 2005, and in 2006 responsibility for implementation was transferred to the Children's Workforce Development Council (CWDC). They were also given the responsibility for developing the skills of all people working with children and young people across all settings (DfES, 2005). The effectiveness of the CAF is still in the early stages, but where coordinated care has been achieved, families have reported a significant improvement in the quality of care (Every Child Matters [ECM], 2007; Department for Children, Schools and Family [DCSF], 2008). See Chapter 3 for further information on the assessment framework and Chapter 6 for the links to parenting.

Research has demonstrated that when a child is cared for at home, there is a shift in emphasis away from illness to recovery and health and there are recommendations that children should not be admitted to hospital unless absolutely necessary (DH/DfES, 2004a; Royal College of Nursing [RCN], 2004). This can only be achieved through coordinated and effective resource management. However, there are many issues around these resources matching the rhetoric of health and social policy.

The Community Children's Nurse (CCN), for example, is trained to work in partnership with the family and other professionals to support children with complex health needs at home, but there are limited numbers of CCNs being trained (RCN 2000). Where there has been good support from the primary care teams, families report a positive outcome and a reduction in hospital visits (RCN, 2000; Chandler, 2007). This requires good communication between all professionals such as the community school nurses, education and other agencies to provide quality care (RCN, 2000; Chandler, 2007). Obviously, if assessment of need is not being realistically addressed, the professional is less likely to be able to influence or empower families to make health promoting changes or choices (see Figure 10.1).

The Expert Patient programme (DH, 2006d) has been introduced to enable individuals and families to gain knowledge and skills about their condition which helps to give them both perceived and actual control over their lives. The expert patient programmes are designed to encourage self-management and the NSF (DH/DfES, 2004a) for children has worked towards tailoring it towards children and young people with complex needs, focusing on the transition processes for adolescents entering adulthood and becoming more independent. This is discussed later.

Theory suggests that having a sense of control will increase the chance of positive health outcomes and encourage changes of behaviour (Kerr *et al.*, 2005). However, this control will depend upon the individual's belief that they can influence the outcomes and this will in turn depend upon their previous experience, their social circumstance, their level of cognition and their self-efficacy (see Figure 10.1). Antonovsky (1996), describing salutogenic theory, considered the construct of a sense of coherence as a mechanism to coping and described three elements to the construct. The first component of coping with adversity was comprehensibility; to understand the world around you and to have the confidence that you can make sense of it. The second component relates to meaningfulness and relates to the concept of seeing positive aspects of their lives and some kind of future. The other element according to Antonovsky is manageability, and this relates to the extent to which families will feel that they have the resources, both material and emotional, to cope with the situation. Although Antonovsky was discussing older people, he also argued that one could apply these concepts to health promotion, and in particular, that building a sense of coherence early in life was a positive strategy. It could also be argued that this is related to self-esteem, and more emphasis in schools to improve self-esteem from an early age, for any child, will enable young people to cope with adversity later in life.

Families, children and young people repeatedly report the frustration of knowing what they require but being confronted by professionals who think they know the family's needs, or who are restricted by funding issues (Sartain *et al.*, 2000; Hewitt-Taylor, 2005). Respite care is one such example with patchy provision and possibly different professionals favouring different types of provision regardless and often in conflict with the family's choice (HM Treasury/DfES, 2007). In addition, the Joseph Rowntree Foundation (2002) reported that black and Asian families in particular are less likely to access community respite care and more likely to struggle alone. This means that these families are marginalised and more likely to enter crisis situations resulting in unnecessary hospital admissions.

Government strategy is to continue the move towards social inclusion, which means supporting children and young people in the community and making the lives of families in difficult circumstances as 'normalised' as possible (DH, 2004; DfES/DH, 2006c). It seems obvious that physical and psychosocial development will be enhanced by creating a sense of normality for these families and there is overwhelming research evidence that well-supported care in the community gives people far better lives than a hospital can. Children who are cared for within their own community benefit from secure emotional and social attachments to family, school and friends (Sartain *et al.*, 2000). Familiar cultural norms and cohesive social relationships create a positive environment for building coping strategies (Hall and Elliman, 2006). The overall impact on the family coping with a complex need can, however, lead to social isolation, poor social networks and family breakdown, and this will inevitably impact on the child's pyscho-social needs.

Children with learning disabilities

According to *Valuing People* (DH, 2001) there were estimated to be around 65,000 children and young people in the UK with a profound or severe learning disability. Learning disabilities are distinct from mental illness or dyslexia as they are lifelong, caused by the way the brain develops before, during or shortly after birth and can be caused by childhood infections or trauma (Mencap, 2007). Children and young people with learning disabilities are defined in *Valuing People* (DH, 2001, p. 21) as having:

A significantly reduced ability to understand new or complex information, to learn new skill (impaired intelligence) with; a reduced ability to cope independently (impaired social function); which started before adulthood with a lasting effect on development.

These are children and families who may require the most support and help with daily living. Many children and young people with learning disabilities also have poor physical and mental health compared to the general population (DH, 2005b; DH, 2007b). For example, people with a learning disability are more likely to have weight problems, both obesity as well as low weight. They are also more prone to some medical conditions than the rest of the population such as spinal problems, epilepsy, respiratory problems, physical disabilities, visual and hearing impairments and dental problems. Research by Mencap has shown that people with a learning disability have a number of unmet health needs (Mencap, 2004). *Valuing People* (DH, 2001), the first White Paper on learning disability for 30 years, outlined the government plan to improve the health of people with learning disabilities in England. There are regular updates on *Valuing People* via the website (Valuing People, 2007).

For young people generally, the transition from adolescence into adulthood is often difficult, and those with a learning disability may be more vulnerable. As carers get older, the future for children with the most profound problems becomes more uncertain and, as they are more likely to be poorer, this creates problems for health and social care services. As young people grow into adulthood, the evidence suggests that unless they have had good support, they are less likely to access health services (Disability Rights Commission [DRC], 2006). The importance, then, of all agencies working together to ensure that specific needs are met in the community, particularly as a child grows up, is vital. The government is committed to closing institutional care and ensuring that people with learning disabilities have opportunities to function within society and not outside it (DH, 2005b, 2007b; HM Treasury/DfES, 2007). Cooperation between education, health, social services and specialist learning disability services will only be successful if the funding through Quality Protects and the Schools Access Initiative is used effectively and efficiently (DH, 2001).

Coordination in the care of children and young people with learning disability will depend upon sustained support from early detection through to the transition into adulthood. Section 312 of the Education Act 1996 (DfES,1996) set out that a child has a special educational need if they have a learning disability that calls for special educational provision to be made. Early intervention is crucial for children with these needs. The inclusion framework set out by Government requires that the needs of children with special educational needs or disabilities are met which includes giving them the opportunity to attend mainstream school (DH/DfES, 2004a). There is a legal framework for this inclusion which sets out clearly the responsibilities of the local authorities, health services and schools in maximising educational opportunities for these children (DfES, 1996; DfES, 2001). Since September 2002, schools have been required to take reasonable steps to ensure that children with disabilities are not placed at a disadvantage to those who are not disabled (DfES, 2001).

There is now more coordination within the early years settings and with schools, which provides a framework for ensuring early detection and support (see Figure 10.2). Early education providers are now inspected by the Office for Standards in Education (Ofsted) and are required to have a Special Education Needs policy (DfES, 2001). Provision in these early years contributes to the overall health and well-being of all children, as it builds on their previous experiences, knowledge, understanding and skills by providing opportunities to develop in six areas of learning (see Table 10.2). For further reading on inclusion see 'Including Me' (Carlin, 2005), a resource providing examples of joint approaches with relevant agencies.

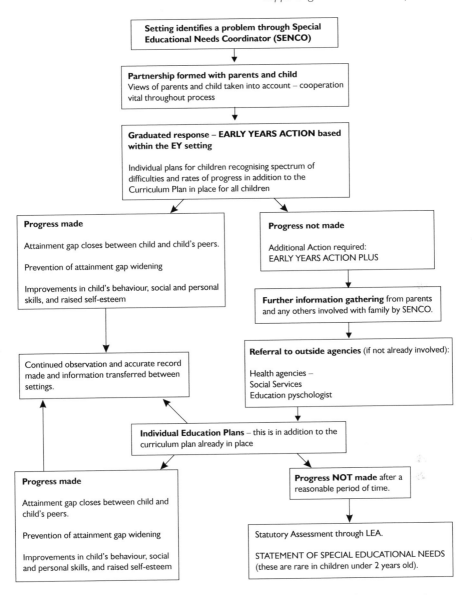

Figure 10.2 Flowchart for referral and support from early years settings.

Learning disability nurses (LDNs) are specifically trained to support children and adults with disabilities, but there are relatively small numbers of them trained and currently working (DH, 2007b). Modernising nursing careers may influence these numbers as role redesign, specialisms and advanced practice are tailored to provide services to meet the specific needs of the population (DH, 2007b). With widening participation and young people living longer into adulthood with complex needs there will need to be consideration of special-

Table 10.2 Early learning goals.

Sets a standard that the majority of children will have achieved by the end of the foundation stage in each of the key learning areas:

- Personal, social and emotional development
- Communication, language and literacy
- Mathematical development
- Knowledge and understanding of the world
- Physical development
- Creative development

(SEN 2001)

NB: This needs to be viewed in the context of the spectrum of learning rates and the range of learning difficulties

ised support across different settings including schools, further education and employment. A good practice guidance on learning disability nursing was published in December 2007 and outlines the importance of specialised services and the value of working in partnership, particularly given the small number of LDNs. Further information on learning disability nursing can also be obtained on the National Network for Learning Disability Nursing (2007).

Children requiring multiple interventions or technical support

Not all children with complex needs will have a disability or special educational needs, but they may have specific medical conditions which also require additional services and technical support; for example, children requiring enteral or parenteral nutrition, ventilatory support or tracheostomy care (see Table 10.1). Children with long-term conditions such as inflammatory bowel disease, cystic fibrosis or asthma will also require consideration in terms of sustained episodes of acute illness, which may continue to require readmission to hospital. Discharge planning should be a top priority on admission to hospital, with good communication between hospital and primary care staff to ensure that children are returned as soon as possible to 'normal' life (Chandler, 2007; Price and Thomas, 2007). There are examples of good cooperation between local authorities and health providers to enable children not only to attend school but also to enjoy activities outside school hours (Carlin, 2005; Brett, 2007). This requires appropriate training to build the confidence of staff in using technology and a willingness to learn. There is also a need to share examples of good practice across the country.

Children with complex medical needs in some areas have increased by up to 39% (Brett, 2007). This may be explained by the advancements in technology, which not only allows children to live longer, but also gives them freedom to be at home, in school and in the community with equipment. The positive aspect of living with more technology is that young people in particular are very familiar with it, using mobile phones, computers and TV as part of their everyday lives. This means that they are more likely to adapt well to the technological advances and feel more able to be a part of society, attend school and enjoy and achieve. Staff involved also need the confidence to work with children and young people out of the comfort zone of the hospital setting. *Modernising Nursing Careers* (DH, 2006b), emphasises the drive to moving care into the community setting and into people's homes. It advocates more flexibility of services, which will require a considered approach to future nurse education (Longley *et al.*, 2007) with more emphasis on the specific skills for working more flexibly across acute and community settings. This includes working with specialised equipment in the home and school environment (RCN, 2001; Carlin, 2000; Brett, 2007). *Modernising Nursing Careers* advocates that careers in the community are a key priority for development (DH, 2006b) and that there will be shifting patterns of service delivery which will require a more creative approach to care. This is also supported by the idea of commissioning services to meet specific need and this will require more effective 'ring fencing' of money for specific areas of need. An area with higher levels of children with life limiting and long-term illnesses (LLIs) and disability may need more community children's nurses, for example (HM Treasury/DfES, 2007). It will also require high levels of cooperation across agencies and settings (Carlin, 2005). There is also recognition of the importance of interprofessional cooperation, extending to interprofessional learning; this is discussed further in Chapter 13.

Consideration of the long-term implications of children with complex needs is vital. This includes examining the transition of adolescents into adulthood, their potential for employment, achieving economic well-being and making a positive contribution (DH, 2004c). The latest report on inequality from *The Equalities Review* (Philips *et al.*, 2007) suggests that at this transitional stage, adolescents with complex needs are at greater risk of not being in education, employment or training. This has a clear impact on their health outcomes and life chances and continues the cycle of inequality. The psychosocial impact of complex needs such as diabetes, inflammatory bowel disease or cystic fibrosis in adolescence has been well documented (WHO, 2007). Adolescents may experience delayed puberty, resent any sense of 'being different' and are more likely to become non-compliant with treatments (WHO, 2007; Harrop, 2007). Becoming a teenager is difficult enough, with the emotional and physical changes, without a complex need as well. The adolescent stage of development is problematic and they report difficulty accessing confidential health services, a lack of accurate information and a failure to respect their views (Royal College of Paediatrics & Child Health [RCPCH], 2003). Those with a complex need may be faced with health professionals who may have known them most of their life and, like parents, they may not be the most appropriate people to support this transition to adulthood. School nurses are in an ideal position to provide emotional support for these young people, as with any other teenager either in the school or home setting, as 'Tier 1' Child and Adolescent Mental Health (CAMHS) support (Lowes, 2007; DfES/DH, 2006). Appropriate management of medical transitions from child to adult service also needs to be addressed and there have long been calls for specialised adolescent services (RCPCH, 2003). There are examples of specialised units across the UK, but these continue to be sporadic in nature and there needs to be a continued effort to provide appropriate resources to offer appropriate services (DH, 2004c).

Social factors

The present Government introduced *Tackling Health Inequalities: A Programme for Action* in July 2003 (DH, 2003), but there continue to be health and social inequalities amongst children and young people and their families (JRF, 2006). For example, infant mortality rates as an indicator vary from 1.6 per 1000 live births in the least deprived areas to 9.8 per 1000 live births in the most deprived areas of the UK (Palmer *et al.*, 2005; DH, 2006c). Although overall child poverty in the UK has fallen over the last ten years, the priorities now are the most disadvantaged, and they make up about 2–3% of the population.

The relationship between complex health needs such as disability and poverty is debated in the literature. Certainly there is evidence to suggest that those with a mental health problem or a learning disability are more likely to fall into that 2–3% of the population (DH, 2007a). Children with complex needs, or children living with parents with a complex need are more likely to be poor due to the difficulties with employment; childcare is expensive, and support networks vary tremendously in individual circumstances (Smith and Middleton, 2007; HM Treasury/DfES, 2007). Increasing the income for these families is important, but there also needs to be an understanding that employment may not necessarily be the complete answer in terms of the child's developmental needs. Certainly, for families coping with a child's complex health needs, employment may not be feasible if they are providing the majority of the care. Accessible child care for these families will allow not only opportunities for earning capacity but also give carers a sense of independence and raise self-esteem (HM Treasury/DfES, 2007).

There is increasing and well-documented evidence of the impact of poverty and social exclusion on children's and young people's health and well-being (DH, 2006c). Children with complex health needs are also often those with complex social needs as well. In 2004 the highest prevalence rates of severely disabled children were among those from semi-skilled manual backgrounds (Office for National Statistics [ONS], 2004) possibly impacting on their economic status. There is also evidence to suggest that there are significant numbers of children from black and other ethnic minorities with complex needs and they are more likely to be living in poverty and less likely to access information and support from statutory bodies (DH, 2007b). Access to quality services has been highlighted in health and social care policies as a key priority (DH, 2006a; HM Treasury/DfES, 2007). Local service level agreements are intended to prioritise service needs, including attention to balancing the care needs of children with their 'disease' needs. *The NSF for Children, Young People and Maternity services: Disabled Children and Young People and Those with Complex Health Needs* (DH/DfES, 2004a) was also introduced to change the way provision of services for children is delivered. This requires a cultural change in the way agencies work together to provide quality care.

There is an intention to provide service models which aim at integrated care, earlier discharges from hospital, reduced hospital admissions and localised services. This provides the overall structural aims of the children's and young people's agenda. The *Children's Workforce Strategy* (DfES, 2005) provides information on the knowledge and skills required by all staff working with children, one of which is that staff strive to reduce inequalities and achieve the best outcomes for children and young people.

This suggests a requirement that all staff working with children have an understanding of public health and health promotion principles and are able to undertake needs assessments (see Chapter 3). It also means that staff need the power to act on this information and therein lies the problem. Many staff recognise problems for both families and populations but often feel powerless to provide solutions due to lack of resources and a lack of funding for public health and health promotion activity (Wanless, 2007). There are some examples of good practice where areas have set up specific services to meet need with good cooperation and team work, but these need sustained resources and commitment by managers, which has not always been the case. Professionals in the teams require skills of building evidence to support the intervention and the means to share models of good practice across the country. This attention to research evidence and improving the skills of the workforce to gather this information has been highlighted for some time and was recognised by the Wanless Report (2007).

In spite of a reduction in overall poverty since 1999, there needs to be recognition that people continue to live in areas of concentrated deprivation with chaotic lifestyles who have fewer opportunities for interaction with others who could provide positive role models for coping strategies (JRF, 2002; DH, 2006c). These hard-to-reach families may fall into the cyclical patterns of behaviour that are well documented. With the drive towards developing public health practitioners (NMC, 2004), there may be a danger that professional individual support will be replaced with a concentration on groups and communities and the truly hard to reach may be marginalised further. *Reaching Out* (DH, 2006c) recognised this and there is acknowledgement that the gaps are continuing to grow for the most disadvantaged people in the UK. Working together from early intervention through school to transition into adulthood is vital (Queens Nursing Institute [QNI], 2007). The Health Visiting review recognised this and advocates intensive home visiting to the most vulnerable families and working in close cooperation with other agencies through to school and beyond (QNI, 2007)

Children as carers

Children who are caring for members of their family with complex needs also need consideration. These children may be coping with very difficult circumstances which can affect their own social, emotional and intellectual development. Some children may be dealing with adult situations and concepts at a very early age, which may mean that they do not have the opportunities for the 'rites of passage' that other children experience – the rebellious teenager for example. The physical and mental health needs of these children may be affected, exhaustion may lead to physical illness, and they are more likely to be living in poverty if family members are unable to work. They may also have more time off school due to caring responsibilities and can be isolated at school or bullied (Young Carers, 2007). The support mechanisms for these children include working in partnership and engagement with the voluntary sector. There is funding from the DfES and DH to support projects aimed at young carers; for example for the Young Carers Initiative, which is a Children's Society project that is working to develop a National Focus for Young Carers, their families and those who work to support them, and to promote common standards and to work towards realising good and equitable services' (Young Carers Initiative, 2008). Continued recognition of the problems these families face is important and school nurses are in a position to support these young people in drop-in services in schools and this must be an area for continuing development (see Chapter 12).

Conclusion

This chapter has outlined some of the issues around promoting the health of children with complex needs. The key to the success, it seems, is to ensure that packages are in place which address individual need and that the most appropriate professionals are working with these families. This will depend upon sustainable resources and assessment of need in the broadest sense of communities but also individual needs in the form of models such as the Common Assessment Framework. It will also require a continuing shift away from traditional care pathways, and an emphasis on effective partnerships. All this has been recognised in the children's agenda but it requires a cultural change within health, social care and education for it to be successful. Working together to achieve health for all children is discussed further in Chapter 13.

References

Antonovsky, A. (1996) The salutogenic model as a theory to guide health promotion. *Health Promotion international,* **11**(1), 11–18.

Brett, J. (2007) Complex needs: improving access to out-of-school activities. *Paediatric Nursing,* **19**(10), 36–9.

Carter, B., Cummings, J. and Cooper, L. (2007) An exploration of best practice in multi-agency working and the experiences of families of children with complex health needs. What works well and what needs to be done to improve practice for the future? *Journal of Clinical Nursing,* **16**(3), 527–39.

Carlin, J. (2005) *Including Me.* The Council for Disabled Children, London.

Chandler, T. (2007) Reducing readmission for asthma: impact of a nurse led service. *Paediatric Nursing,* **19**(10), 19–21.

Davidson, L. (2003) *Health Systems in the United Kingdom and Their Role in Increasing Equity.* http://www.pediatrics.org/; accessed 2 July 2007.

Debell, D. (ed.) (2007) *Public Health Practice and the School Age Population.* Edward Arnold, London.

Department for Education and Skills (DfES) (1996) *The Education Act.* DfES, London.

Department for Education and Skills (2001) *Special Educational Needs: Code of Practice.* DfES, London.

Department for Education and Skills (2005) *Children's Workforce Strategy: a Strategy to Build A World-class Workforce for Children and Young People.* DfES, London.

Department for Education and Skills/Department of Health (2006) *School Nurse: Practice Development Resource Pack.* DfES, London.

Department for Children, Schools and Families (2008). Research (services for children). http://www.dfes.gov.uk/research/; accessed 8 January 2008.

Department of Health (2000) *The Framework for Assessment of Children in Need*. Stationery Office, London.

Department of Health (2001) *Valuing People*. Stationery Office, London.

Department of Health (2003) *Tackling Health Inequalities: a Programme for Action*. DH, London.

Department of Health (2004) *Practice Based Commissioning: Promoting Clinical Engagement*. DH, London.

Department of Health (2005a) *Making Practice Based Commissioning a Reality: Technical Guidance*. DH, London.

Department of Health (2005b) *The Government's Annual Report on Learning Disability*. Stationery Office, London.

Department of Health (2006a) *Our Health Our Care Our Say*. Stationery Office, London.

Department of Health (2006b) *Modernising Nursing Careers*. DH, London.

Department of Health (2006c) *The Expert Patient Programme; a New Approach to Disease Management for the 21st Century*. DH, London.

Department of Health (2007a) *Progress on Social Exclusion*. DH, London.

Department of Health (2007b) *Good Practice in Learning Disability Nursing*. DH, London.

Department of Health, Department for Education and Skills (2004a) *National Service Framework for Children, Young People and Maternity Services: Disabled Children and Young People and Those with Complex Health Needs*. DH, London.

Department of Health, Department for Education and Skills (2004b) *National Service Framework for Children, Young People and Maternity Services: Executive Summary*. DH, London.

Department for Work and Pensions (2006) *The Family Resources Survey*. DWP, London.

Department for Work and Pensions (2007) *Working for Children*. DWP, London.

Disability Rights Commission (2006) *Report on the DRC Formal Inquiry Panel to the DRC's Formal Investigation into the Inequalities in Physical Health Experienced by People with Mental Health Problems and People with Learning Disabilities*. DRC, London

Every Child Matters (2007) Common Assessment Framework. http://www.everychild-matters.gov.uk/deliveringservices/caf/; accessed 8 January 2008.

Hall, D. and Elliman, D. (2006) *Health for all Children*, 4th edn. Oxford University Press, Oxford.

Harrop, M. (2007) Psychosocial impact of cystic fibrosis in adolescence. *Paediatric Nursing*, **19**(10), 41–5.

HM Government (2006) *Reaching Out: an Action Plan on Social Exclusion*. HM Government and Social Exclusion Unit, London.

Hewitt-Taylor, J. (2005) Caring for children with complex and continuing health needs. *Nursing Standard*, **19**(42), 41–7.

Hodgkinson, R. and Lester, H. (2002) Stresses and coping strategies of mothers living with a child with cystic fibrosis: implications for nursing professionals. *Journal of Advanced Nursing*, **39**(4), 377–83.

HM Treasury/DfES (2007) *Aiming High for Disabled Children: Better Support for Families*. Office of Public Sector Information, Norwich.

Joseph Rowntree Foundation (2002) Providing better access to short breaks for black disabled children and their parents. http://www.jrf.org,uk/knowledge/findings/socialcare/582.asp; accessed 27 November 2007.

Joseph Rowntree Foundation (2006) *What Will it Take to End Child Poverty?* http://www.jrf.org.uk/knowledge/findings/socialpolicy/0366.asp; accessed 3 January 2008.

Kerr, J., Weitunat, R. and Moretti, M. (2005) *ABC of Behaviour Change: a Guide to Successful Disease Prevention and Health Promotion*. Elsevier Churchill Livingstone, London.

Longley, M., Shaw, C., Dolan, G. and Stackhouse, R. (2007) *Nursing: Towards 2015*. Commissioned by the NMC – Welsh Institute for Health and Social Care, University of Glamorgan, Pontypridd, Wales.

Lowes, L. (2007) Impact on child and family. In: *Nursing Care of Children and Young People with Chronic Illness* (eds. F. Valentine and L. Lowes). Blackwell Publishing, Oxford.

Mencap (2004) *Treat Me Right: Better Healthcare for People with Learning Disabilities*. Mencap, London.

Mencap (2007) *What Causes Disability?* http://www.mencap.org.uk/html/about_learning_disability/learning_disability_causes.asp; accessed 1 December 2007.

Nursing and Midwifery Council (2004) *Standards of Proficiency for Specialist Community Public Health Nurses*. NMC, London.

Office for National Statistics (2004) *The Health of Children and Young People: Disability*. http://www.statistics.gov.uk/cci/nugget.asp?id=795; accessed 8 January 2008.

Palmer, G., Carr, J. and Kenway, P. (2005) *Monitoring Poverty and Social Exclusion in the UK*. Joseph Rowntree Foundation, London.

Peate, I. and Whiting, L. (eds.) (2006) *Caring for Children and Families*. John Wiley & Sons, Chichester.

Philips, R. K., Kerslake, R. and Mayhew, J. (2007) *Fairness and Freedom: the Final Report of the Equalities Review: a Summary*. The Equalities Review, London.

Price, M. and Thomas, S. (2007) Continuing care needs. In: *Nursing Care of Children and Young People with Chronic Illness* (eds. F. Valentine and L. Lowes). Blackwell Publishing, Oxford.

Queen's Nursing Institute (2007) *Facing the Future; a Review of the Role of the Health Visitor*. QNI, London.

Royal College of Paediatric and Child Health (2003) *Bridging the Gaps: Health Care for Adolescents*. RCPCH, London.

Royal College of Nursing (2000) *Children's Community Nursing: Promoting Effective Teamworking for Children and Their Families*. RCN, London.

Royal College of Nursing (2001) *Administering Intravenous Therapy to Children in the Community Setting*. RCN, London.

Royal College of Nursing (2004) *Commissioning Health Care Services for Children and Young People: Increasing Nurses' Influence*. RCN, London.

Sartain, S., Clarke, C. and Heyman, R. (2000) Hearing the voices of children with a chronic illness. *Journal of Advanced Nursing*, **32**(4), 913–21.

Sidell, M., Jones, L., Katz, J., Peberdy, A. and Douglas, J. (eds.) *Debates and Dilemmas in Promoting Health*. Palgrave Macmillan, London.

Smith, N. and Middleton, S. (2007) *Poverty Dynamics Research in the UK*. Joseph Rowntree Foundation, London.

Valentine, F. and Lowes, L. (2007) *Nursing Care of Children and Young People with Chronic Illness*. Blackwell Publishing, Oxford.

Valuing People (2007) http://valuingpeople.gov.uk/index.jsp; accessed 3 January 2008.

Wanless, D. (2002) *Securing Our Future Health: Taking a Long-Term View*. HM Treasury, London.

Wanless, D. (2007) *Our Future Health Secured? A Review of NHS Funding and Performance*. King's Fund Publications, London.

World Health Organization (2007) *The Adolescent with a Chronic Condition; Epidemiology, Developmental Issues and Health Care Provision*. http://www.who.int/; accessed 3 January 2008.

Young Carers (2007) *Gemma's Story*. http://www.youngcarers.net/; accessed 3 January 2008.

Young Carers Initiative (2008) http://www.youngcarer.com/showPage.php?file=initiative.htm; accessed 8 January 2008.

Useful websites

Connexions: http://www.connexions-tw.co.uk/

Joseph Rowntree Foundation: http://www.jrf.org.uk/

The King's Fund: http://www.kingsfund.org.uk/

Valuing People: http://www.valuingpeople.gov.uk/

The National Children's Bureau: http://www.ncb.org.uk/Page.asp

National Network for Learning Disability: http://www.nnldn.org.uk/

National Institute for Clinical Health Excellence: http://www.nice.org.uk/

CHAPTER 11

Safeguarding the health of children and young people in public care

Maxine Jameson

Key themes

- Who are the children in public care in England?
- Legislative framework to promote the health of children in the care system
- The health needs of children in care
- Working with children and young people who are looked after

Health needs of looked after children: who are looked after children?

Children and young people looked after away from home may be:

- Accommodated under a voluntary agreement with their parent(s) consent, or their own consent if aged 16 or 17
- In care on a Care Order or interim Care Order under Section 31 of the Children Act 1989
- Accommodated under Section 21(2)(C)(I) of the Children Act 1989 (remanded to Local Authority care)
- On an Emergency Protection Order under Section 44 of the Children Act 1989

Children enter the care system for a variety of reasons, most have experienced parental neglect or abuse and 66% are looked after under court orders.

While the majority of children are looked after by foster carers, there is a growing trend for children to be subject to a care order by living at home or placed with family friends approved as foster carers. A minority of children, 13%, live in residential homes. Almost uniquely these are older children, only 2% of children in residential care are under 10 years of age. An important overall trend is that children are entering care at a younger age and staying for longer periods (DfES, 2006). At any one point in time about 60,000 children are looked after by local authorities in England and Wales. More than half the population of looked after children are over 10; this group includes those children who have grown up in care and older children entering the system. The majority of children spend only a brief period of time in the care system, but about a fifth remain in care on a long-term basis. Very few of these children will move into the security of an adoptive family. In 2006, only 3,700 children were adopted from the care system (DfES, 2006).

Introduction

Children and young people who are looked after by the local authority include all those children provided with accommodation as part of a voluntary arrangement with the child's carers as well as those children formally in the care of local authority as part of a voluntary order of the court, these children are amongst the most socially excluded groups in England and Wales. They have increased health needs in comparison with children and young people from comparable socio-economic backgrounds who have not needed to be taken into care, and these needs often remain unmet (Chambers *et al.*, 2002). As a result, many children and young people who are looked after experience significant health inequalities and on leaving care experience very poor health, educational and social outcomes (Department of Health, 2002). The physical and mental health of children in care is often poor in comparison to that of their peers with higher levels of substance misuse, significantly higher rates of teenage pregnancy and a much greater prevalence of mental health problems (Chambers, 2002). Absence of birth parents often leads to distress and destructive ways of coping, including violence and criminal behaviour (Hill, 2003).

The poor physical and mental state of children and young people in care has concerned practitioners and policy makers for many years. It was hoped that the Children Act 1989 would significantly improve the health outcomes for children in care. This Act placed great emphasis on preventative work with children and families. However, a series of later reports suggested that improvements in health indicators and outcomes have failed to materialise (Utting, 1997; Acheson, 1998; Skuse and Ward, 1999; Wyler, 2000).

With such strong evidence that the needs of looked after children were remaining unaddressed, the Department of Health (DfES, 2006) launched new guidelines *Promoting the Health of Looked After Children* (DH, 2002). This guidance sets out a framework for the delivery of services from health agencies and local councils, with social services' responsibilities designed to promote and improve the health of looked after children and young people. The guidance set out to: 'support the development of an effective and flexible system which will address health inequalities and the assessment of health needs, obtain and manage the information required to produce individual health plans for all looked after children and young people and enable these plans to be implemented' (p. 177). The guidance provided a set of underpinning principles on which the service should be based and outlines key roles and responsibilities for relevant agencies. It gave a framework for the delivery of services and outlined three areas where improvement and change were required:

- The development of an effective and flexible system which would address the inequalities and the assessment of health needs, obtain and manage the information required to produce individual health care plans for all looked after children and young people.
- A set of underpinning principles on which services should be based and outlines key roles and responsibilities of all relevant agencies.
- A shift away from a health care system based on annual medicals towards a more holistic assessment of an individual child and young person's health care needs.

Much of the literature concerned with the health of looked after children and young people relates to accounts of ill health (Mather and Batty, 2000). The past focus has been upon identifying and reducing illness through medical interventions. In the past the system of yearly medical checks left young people feeling 'processed' without achieving the desired result of improved health and care. The latest guidance from the Department of Health, outlined above, reflected a radical commitment to a more holistic model of health care, one concerned with far more than the absence of illness. It has been recognised that, to be successful, health improvement programmes require the active participation and empowerment of young people as primary custodians of their own health. Looked after children's nurses and doctors are now encouraged to listen to children and young people and involve them in the development and delivery of the service. This is quite a change in service provision and can be interpreted by professionals in differing ways across the country.

Hill (2003, p. 343) suggests: 'We do not know enough about the effectiveness in terms of outcomes of involving children and young people in agenda setting, however, evidence from other areas of healthcare suggest that a user-driven agenda makes for services which are more accessible and acceptable'. Such a statement called for more research in this area and it highlights the need to find out what the felt needs of children who are looked after are.

Legislative framework

All services in place to support looked after children are underpinned by the principles contained in the United Nations Convention on the Rights of the Child (UNICEF,1991), which was ratified by the UK Government in 1991, the Children Act (DH 1989: DH, 2004) and The Care Standards Act (2000).

The key issues are highlighted in the following articles:

- *Article 3*: the best interests of the child should be a primary consideration when action is taken concerning children.
- *Article 24*: the rights of any child to the enjoyment of the highest attainable standard of health and to facilities for the treatment of illness and the rehabilitation of health.
- *Article 25*: the right of the child placed by competent authorities for the purpose of care protection or treatment of his mental or physical health, to a periodic review of the treatment provided to the child and all other circumstances relevant to his placement.
- *Article 39*: all appropriate measures to be taken to promote the physical and psychological recovery and social reintegration of a child victim of any form of abuse or neglect.

The Children Act (DH, 2004) provides a comprehensive framework for the care and protection of all children and young people in need. Local authorities have a specific duty to safeguard and promote the well-being of children looked after by them. This legislation places specific duties on councils with social service responsibilities to promote the health of looked after children. In 2002, amendments to the Children Act were made (Children Act Miscellaneous Amendments (England) Regulations 20) in view of the evidence of high levels of unmet need to this population. The revised framework, *Promoting the Health of Looked After Children* (Department of Health 2002) is significant for the health of young people. The key changes are:

- The first health assessment is required to be undertaken by an appropriately qualified registered medical practitioner.
- Review assessments may be carried out by an appropriately qualified nurse/midwife.

■ The requirements for a local authority health assessment on children aged under 5 are now twice yearly.

The state as a substitute parent

All children have the right to the highest attainable standards of health and facilities for treatment (UNICEF, 1991). Childhood is a period of continuous growth and development and most parents aim from the time their children are born to promote physical, emotional, social and psychological growth. Children who cannot be brought up by their birth parents have the same rights as other children. So how does the state perform as a substitute parent? In 2006, 26% of young people in accommodation aged 14–16 years were excluded from or not attending education, between 50% and 75% of young people leaving care had no academic qualifications compared with 6% of the general population and less than 19% continued in further education compared to 66% of the general population (DfES, 2006). In addition, 66% of looked after young people had mental health problems compared with 15% of the population, while 23% had major depressive illness compared with 4% of the population and 14% of looked after girls were pregnant or had babies while in the care system or within a year of leaving. A national drug and alcohol survey found 44% of substance abusers had been in care, a third of whom had started abusing substances whilst being looked after, and that 50% of young people were living rough (DfES, 2006a). Twenty three per cent of adult prisoners and 38% of young prisoners have been in care (DfES, 2006a). Although outcomes for children in care have improved in recent years, there remains a significant and widening gap between outcomes for children in care and outcomes for all children.

Health needs of looked after children

A series of Government reports have highlighted the health neglect, unhealthy lifestyles and mental health needs that characterise children and young people living in care. Looked after children epitomise the 'inverse care law' whereby those with the worst health get the least treatment; their health needs may not only be jeopardised by abusive and neglectful parenting, but care itself may fail to repair and protect health. Indeed, it may even exacerbate damage and abuse.

Children with disabilities and learning difficulties are over-represented in the looked after children population (DfES, 2006a). Many have suffered emotional, sexual or physical abuse. Some are looked after because of risks posed by their parents' lifestyles. This has implications for their own health; for example, children suffering from the effects of alcohol or drug abuse during pregnancy and those born to parents suffering from genetic conditions that have health implications for the children (Turnpenny, 1995). Children from ethnic minority backgrounds suffer particular discrimination, but until recently national statistics were not kept on the ethnicity of looked after children. Many looked after children from all backgrounds have experienced interrupted or damaged attachment patterns in their early lives and will have continuing attachment difficulties. Some have a range of behavioural difficulties arising from their early experiences or because of their specific needs (Jewett, 1995). Before coming into care, looked after children's health has often been compromised by poverty, poor diet or poor housing. Many children will have missed routine child health surveillance, regular vision and dental checks. Immunisation uptake may be poor; absence or exclusion from school produces educational failure, which further impacts on health. Particularly important is the damage to the child's coping mechanism and self-esteem caused by inconsistent and poor parenting. Low self-esteem makes it extremely difficult for children to take responsibility for their own health and lifestyle.

Many looked after children experience frequent changes of carer and school; change of social worker further damages continuity. Poor record keeping and the delayed transmission of health records compound this situation. There may be no previous medical records, thus encouraging over-reliance on isolated and uncoordinated medical examinations. Many children are not registered with a GP; poor communications between health and social services leads to confusion about who is responsible for action. There can be difficulty in obtaining consent for medical treatment with a lack of clarity as to who can give consent, the parent, the foster carer, the local authority or even the young person.

History of looked after children's health assessments

Until the 1960s looked after children had to undergo Freedom From Infection (FFI) inspections. The child, invariably accompanied by a social worker, who knew little about them, would be undressed, checked for bruises and infestations and duly declared 'free from infection'. This procedure did nothing for the child or his dignity, and has been abandoned. However, the contrast between arrangements for children living with their families and those fostered and in residential care continues. The looked after child is often only registered as a temporary patient with the foster carer's general practitioner. Thus the child receives acute or urgent treatment, but the preventative care, health surveillance and immunisation offered to every other child is effectively denied to those most in need. Serious undiagnosed problems continue to be found in pre-adoption medical checks carried out on children who have spent many years in care (Mather *et al.*, 1997b; DfES, 2007).

It is now a statutory requirement (DH, 2002) that all children in the care system should have a medical examination carried out by a registered medical practitioner within one month of the child's entry into the care system. The regulatory framework provides for an annual health assessment for each child or young person over five who is looked after (six monthly for children under 5 years). The objective of these arrangements is to ensure that health needs are properly addressed and appropriate health care interventions provided. Historically, however, the coverage of these assessments has been patchy, with large regional variations (DH, 2002).

Health assessments have been regarded as annual 'medicals' with undue emphasis on the performing of a physical examination and inadequate attention paid to personal history. Issues such as health promotion and the concerns of the children and young people themselves have often been overlooked.

When health assessments do take place they frequently identify the need for investigation or specialist referral. However, looked after children experience frequent moves in and out of the care system or between a series of placements. During 2000, 18% of looked after children moved between three or more placements (DH, 2002) increased mobility means that health care decisions tend not to be implemented or to be seriously delayed.

A health care system based on annual 'medicals' has made many children and young people feel disengaged from their own health issues. A survey by the Who Cares? Trust showed that 40% of looked after children under 11 felt that they had not received enough health information and advice, and around half of those in children's homes and secure units considered that they had put their own health at risk in some way (Who Cares? Trust, 1998). McGuire and Corlyon (1997) found that the requirement to have an annual 'medical' is regarded as stigmatising by many children and young people and this leads many to refuse to attend.

It is hoped that the introduction of the latest legislation *Promoting the Health of Looked After Children* (DH, 2002; DfES, 2007), will achieve a shift away from the medical model of health care and towards a more holistic assessment of need. It aims for a system that works with, not for, children and empowers both children and young people to make informed decisions about their own health.

Safeguarding the health of looked after children

For the past 30 years statutory annual medical examination was often viewed as the principal safeguard for the health of looked after children. The 'Freedom From Infection' examination emphasised the need to protect the health of the foster carer families rather than promote the health of the child. In England and Wales the 1991 regulations of the Children Act (1989) emphasised the health rather than the social dimensions of the health check by stipulating that the examination should be undertaken by a 'registered medical practitioner'. A medical approach was further encouraged by the format of the British Adoption and Fostering forms that are used to complete health examinations; these forms focus mainly on the medical examination and physical development of the child.

Problems with medical checks

Large studies in the 1990s suggest that statutory medicals were poorly attended, with uptake rates of 25% and below (Butler and Payne, 1997; Mather *et al.*, 1997b). When reasons for poor uptake were explored young people expressed negative views of the process: 'Having to take your clothes off for a strange doctor when you don't feel ill is yet one more abuse of the system'. (Mather and Batty, 2000, pp. 221–6). Policy developments have sought to address these difficulties. The growing evidence of health neglect and disadvantage in the population of looked after children was highlighted by a UK Parliamentary review (House of Commons Committee, 1998) which recommended a new approach to promoting the health of looked after children. This was followed by Department of Health Guidelines for Looked After Children (2002). These guidelines recognised the place for health assessments rather than medical assessments, and encouraged a move a way from the medical model to a more flexible and holistic assessment. In this guidance the role of health profession-als other than doctors is promoted.

In April 2002 amendments to the Arrangements of Placements of Children Regulations (in the Children Act, 1989) permitted registered nurses and mid-wives, under the supervision of a doctor, to undertake review health assess-ments. This shift in policy created an opportunity for many health trusts and local authorities to employ nurses to enhance the health of looked after chil-dren. Until recently there has been no evidence of any systematic monitoring of health progress and outcomes in looked after children; it is also difficult to distinguish between problems proceeding or consequent to the child's care experiences.

Children and young people suffer poor emotional health often due to many placement changes, loneliness, isolation and low-self esteem. Evidence suggests that children often are not listened to and are unable to develop long-lasting relationships due to the frequent moves they make whilst in care.

Poor attendance at school is a strong theme in the discussion of children in care, with between half and three quarters of children leaving care with no qualifications, resulting in over half of teenagers leaving care unemployed, thus continuing the circle of deprivation long after they have left the care system. In 2006 only 7% of children in care obtained 5 GCSEs (DfES, 2006a), considerably lower than results obtained by young people generally.

Children and young people who are looked after are reported to have greater physical health needs than their peers, yet are less likely to receive adequate health care and treatment often due to poor attendance rates (often as low as 25%) at health check-ups, (Butler, 1997; Cleaver, 1997). Hill *et al.* (2002) suggested that when they do attend they often receive a disease screening exercise rather than health promotion.

Looked after children need to be supported in developing their knowledge and skills in making decisions that promote health and well-being. There needs to be an emphasis on the need for a holistic approach to health care and that improved inter-agency working is key to the development of services for children in care.

> For too long society has failed children in care and it is nothing less than a scandal. We should have the same aspirations for these children as we do our own (Alan Johnson, Education Secretary: ECM, 2007a).

Health professionals and social workers both acknowledge that the present systems of care are failing looked after children. There remains serious failures to communicate a major issue between social services and health. Butler and Payne (1997), Grant *et al.* (2002) and Hill and Watkins (2003) all recommended that health assessments should be complementary to and integrated with local authority care and review if they are to be successful. This recommendation has since been taken forward by the Department of Health (2002) but has yet to be implemented by many Primary Care Trusts.

The Green Paper *Care Matters: Transforming the Lives of Children and Young People in Care* (DfES, 2005b) set out priorities for change for PCTs and states that the childhood we are giving looked after children has not been good enough. 'The time has come to accelerate the pace of change, and to make care not only a way out of difficult situations at home, but a bridge to better childhood and a better future' (p. 48). A lot of progress has been made over the last decade in improving outcomes for children generally; we have seen an increase of eleven percentage points in the proportion of all young people gaining 5 A*–C GCSEs and the proportion of young people in education, employment or training by 19 now stands at 87% – the highest it has ever been. This progress needs to be replicated with young people in care.

In line with reforms for children's services through the Every Child Matters (DfES, 2004) programme, PCTs are encouraged to identify problems early and respond to them quickly by offering sustained and multidisciplinary support. Public sector agreements have set two targets to improve outcomes for looked after children, improving the stability of their placements and improving their educational outcomes, to support the delivery of these targets the government is working closely with local authorities to ensure that their policies and practices support placement stability (ECM, 2007b). The introduction of some financial support should facilitate the working together of PCTs, local authorities and Children's Trusts.

Children in care are a group who are especially deserving of our help precisely because they are in care. 'As their corporate parent the State cannot and must not accept any less for them than we would for our own children' (Care Matters, 2006). Policy reform and the setting of targets are a starting point; the implementation by different health and social care workers and organisations should make this a reality.

To improve life chances of children in care the following are necessary:

- The introduction of holistic health assessments. There is a general view that the system is 'processing' young people without achieving the desired result of improved health and care. There is the need for a reassessment of health care with the introduction of nurse led reviews.
- Integrated care between local authorities and health and improved communication systems.
- A reduction in the number of placement changes experienced by children which adversely effects the emotional health of the child.
- Looked after children need a stable home and an adult to champion their cause.
- A stable and quality education is paramount if we are to give looked after children equal life chances.

Conclusion

This chapter has explored the issues surrounding children and young people looked after by the State. It has examined the history of the care system and has presented key research evidence as to why looked after children present a significant public health concern. Those working with such children must be knowledgeable about the new legislative and multi-agency practice issues surrounding looked after children and the implications this has for practice if they are to improve life chances for this vulnerable group. These children need a stable home, quality education and a designated professional to champion their cause.

Adopting an holistic approach is crucial in ensuring that looked after children get the best possible care. Only by good collaborative working and improved communications across disciplines can we begin to reduce the inequalities looked after children face.

References

Acheson, D. (1998) *Independent Inquiry into Inequalities in Health*. Stationery Office, London.

Butler, I. and Payne, H. (1997) The health of children looked after by local authority. *Adoption and Fostering*, **21**(2), 28–35.

Chambers, H., Howell, S., Madge, N. and Olle, H. (2002) *Healthy Care*. National Children's Bureau, London.

Cleaver. H. (1997) New research on teenagers. Key findings and the implications on practice. *Adoption and Fostering*, **21**(1), 37–43.

Department for Education and Skills (2004) *Every Child Matters: Next Steps*. DfES Publications, Nottingham.

Department for Education and Skills (2006a) *Children Looked after in England 2005–6*. DfES Publications, Nottingham.

Department for Education and Skills (2006b) *Care Matters: Transforming the Lives of Children and Young People in Care*. Stationery Office, London.

Department for Education and Skills (2007) *Care Matters*. DfES, London. http://www.everychildmatters.gov.uk/socialcare/lookedafterchildren/; accessed 22 September 2007.

Department of Health (1998) *Caring for Children Away from Home, Messages From Research*. Wiley, Chichester.

Department of Health (2002) *Promoting the Health of Looked After Children*. Department of Health, London.

Every Child Matters (2007a) *Looked After Children*. Care Matters White Paper launched, Press release. http://www.everychildmatters.gov.uk/socialcare/lookedafterchildren/?asset=News&id=67202; accessed 21 January 2008.

Every Child Matters (2007b) *Looked After Children*. http://www.everychildmatters.gov.uk/socialcare/lookedafterchildren/; accessed 21 January 2008.

Gallagher, B. (1999) The abuse of children in public care. *Child Abuse Review*, 357–5.

Grant, A., Ennis, J. and Stuart, F. (2002) Looking after health: a joint working approach to improving the health of looked after and accommodated children and young people. *Scottish Journal of Residential Care*, **1**, 23–8.

Hall, D. and Elliman, D. (2003) *Health for All Children*. Oxford University Press, Oxford.

Hill, C. and Watkins, J. (2003) Statutory Health Assessments for looked-after children: what do they achieve? *Child Care, Health and Development*, **29**(1), 3–13.

Hill, C., Wright, V., Sampeys, C., Dunnett, K., Daniel, S., O'Dell, L. and Watkins, J. (2002) The emerging role of the specialist nurse, promoting the health of looked after children. *Adoption and Fostering*, **26**(4), 35–43.

House of Commons Select Committee on Health (1998) *Children Looked After by Local Authorities (Second Report)*. House of Commons Publications, London.

House of Commons (1998) *The Health of Children Looked After by Local Authorities*. Report by the Department of Health Select Committee. HMSO, London.

Howell, S. (2001) *Promoting Health in Care: a Literature Review. National Healthy Care Standard*. National Children's Bureau, London.

Jewett, G. (1995) *Helping Children Cope with Separation and Loss*. BAAF, London.

Kahan, B. (1989) The physical and mental health of children in care. In *Child Care Research, Policy and Practice* (ed. B. Kahan). Hodder & Stoughton/Open University, London.

Mather, M. and Batty, D. (2000) *Doctors for Children in Public Care*. British Agencies for Adoption and Fostering, London.

Mather, M., Humphrey, J. and Robson, J. (1997a) The statutory medical and health needs of looked after children. *Adoption and Fostering*, **21**, 2.

Mather, M., Humphrey, J. and Robson, J. (1997b) The statutory medical and health needs of looked after children. Time for a radical review? *Adoption and Fostering*, **21**, 36–40.

McGuire, C. and Corlyon, J. (1997) *Health Promotion and Looked After Children in Brent and Harrow*. National Children's Bureau, London.

Skuse, T. and Ward, H. (1999) *Looking After Children, the Final Report to the Department of Health*. Loughborough University, Loughborough.

Turnpenny, P. (1995) *Secrets in the Genes*. BAAF. London.

UNICEF (1991) *United Nations Convention on the Rights of the Child*, January 1991. http://www.unicef.org/.

Utting, W. (1991) *Children in the Public Care: A Review of Residential Care*. SSI/HMSO, London.

Who Cares? Trust (1998) *Remember My Message*. Who Cares? Trust, London.

Wyler, S. (2000) *The Health of Young People Leaving Care: a Review for the King's Fund/Oak Foundation*. King's Fund, London.

Resources

Champions for Children and Young People in Care can be contacted via the Community Practitioners and Health Visitors Association in London; Tel 020 7939 7000.

CHAPTER 12

Children out of the school setting

Ros Godson

Key themes

- Children and young people are out of the school setting for many different reasons
- They do not form a homogeneous group
- Such children and young people have a variety of health, social and educational needs
- Health and other workers together with the wide society are, or should be, active in promoting their well-being

Introduction

Responsibility for a child's education rests with the parents. However, although education is compulsory from age 5 to 16 years in England, schooling is not. Parents can elect to educate their children at home, and take financial responsibility for giving 'an efficient education, suitable to the age, ability and aptitude of the child'. (Education Act 1996: section 7)

Universal primary education is one of the eight UN Millennium Development Goals (2000), as it is recognised that education of parents is one way to improve the health and well-being of the next generation. Compulsory education is seen as critical for a child's future life chances. Indeed, for many children from chaotic backgrounds, school is a place of safety where they can attain qualifications to improve their prospects and experience stability and a consistent approach to life. Those who do not attend are in danger of becoming involved in risk-taking behaviour and criminality. The MORI youth survey (2004) showed that nearly half of those in mainstream education who had committed an offence said they had played truant from school and three quarters of excluded pupils who had committed an offence had also played truant. Many young people suffer temporary setbacks and can be helped by parents and school; however, for some young people, an accumulation of problems overwhelms their resources, and problems can become severe and entrenched. The five outcomes from Every Child Matters (2004) are relevant to all children and young people, and particular initiatives have been set in place to tackle teenage pregnancy, substance misuse, anti-social behaviour and youth crime.

Exclusions and truancy

The Department for Education and Skills data indicates that in excess of 9,000 pupils are permanently excluded from school each year, and up to 10,000 pupils are missing from school completely (Ofsted, 2004). In addition, authorised and unauthorised absence from school accounts for approximately 9% of total school days. English national targets and initiatives have been introduced to improve the support for those pupils at risk of becoming disaffected or excluded (Ofsted, 2004). The Scottish government reports that on average there are 48,000 pupil days missed (7%), of which 22,200 are due to sickness, 5,600 to truanting, 3,600 to holidays and about 800 to temporary exclusion (Scottish Government News, 2007).

In Northern Ireland there were approximately 4,500 days when children were out of school across all age ranges, but this increases markedly at secondary level (Department of Education, 2006).

There are many reasons why children and young people are not in school, a TUC report in 2001 (TUC, 2001) found that 10% children admitted truanting in order to carry out paid work. This may be doing paper rounds or helping in the family business, babysitting or cleaning. Of these children, 25% reported being too tired to attempt all of their school work and homework. This is obviously against the law and local authorities are obliged to act upon information received (DCSF, 2007a). Children who do not attend school miss out on extra curricular activities as well as educational ones, which potentially impacts on their physical and social development.

The Children's Plan (DCSF, 2007b) acknowledges that once a pupil is excluded from mainstream school, their chances of acquiring a decent education may be severely curtailed, owing to variability in the quality of services which can be offered by the local education department. The Children's Plan talks of the alternative of 'studio schools' which will offer more vocational education, and be linked to local businesses.

Education otherwise

It is not clear how many children are educated outside of the school system, as there is no mechanism to record this. A small study (Hopwood *et al.*, 2007) commissioned by the Department for Education and Skills suggested that 0.09% to 0.42% of the total school aged population are electively home educated. This equates to between 1 in 237 and 1 in 1,133 children being educated at home.

The study indicates that equal numbers of girls and boys are in home education and twice as many at secondary level than primary. Some education authorities have robust systems to make sure that children are not 'lost' to the school system at transition to secondary school. There may be a slightly higher than average number of children with special educational needs. This option is taken up by Roma, gypsy, and traveller groups as well as indigenous families. Reasons for home education vary from religious, cultural or ideological beliefs to dissatisfaction with the quality of education at school or bullying. For some this is a very positive experience when parents or carers believe, sometimes with justification, that the local schools cannot meet the needs of their child.

Yet, there is a dilemma here for local education authorities who have a duty to ensure that adequate education is being provided to every child, and that the child's welfare and safety are ensured. Parents can prevent the local authority from entering their home or seeing the child. If they have good reason to think that a child is not receiving suitable education, then they can issue a written notice requiring parents to engage with education staff; if they refuse, the local authority can serve a School Attendance Order (SAO).

Young carers

The 2001 census found there were 150,000 young carers in England and Wales, defined as under 18 year olds who provide personal or health care to another family member (often their mother) on a regular basis (Dearden and Becker, 1998). Although this is more likely in a lone parent household, it does not mean that children in two-parent households are never carers. This duty is physically and emotionally draining for the young person, and they may have difficulties with doing homework, maintaining friendships, taking part in leisure activities, and sometimes missing or being late for school. The plight of these children and young people has become better understood in the last few years. Dearden and Becker's report (2004) found that still 22% of young carers fail to access all of their education. This can mean that they miss out on vital opportunities and career choices. Children caring for someone with drug or alcohol problems were significantly more likely to have problems accessing education.

It is important that school staff understand the difficulties that these pupils may have, as otherwise the stress on them is exacerbated. They may need to ring home during the day, or defer school work. They may be unable to attend after-school activities or go on school cultural trips. Caring is demanding but not always consistent; there may be busy nights, when the young person is too tired for school work the next day. Good liaison with the school nurse will facilitate understanding and support, as the young person may have frequent concerns and questions about their patient's health, medicine and prognosis.

The Community Care (Scotland) Act, 2002 extended the rights to an assessment to all young carers providing 'regular and significant care', in addition to the needs of the client, and the Children Act (1989) did the same in England and Wales. Many young people are proud of the care they give, and although they welcome outside agencies' help, they can be quite specific about what is needed, and may not want to give up all their duties.

Special educational needs

Children with special education needs should normally be educated in mainstream schools where that is the wish of the parents, and suitable education must be provided. Where mainstream school is considered inappropriate, perhaps because of the child's condition, then alternative provision, acceptable to the child's parents, must be offered by the education authority (Education Act 1996). Disputes sometimes arise when the education authority refuses to fund a particular provision which the parents think is suitable for their child, but where the education authority insists that a local mainstream or special school can provide satisfactory education. This can lead to parents keeping their child away from school during an appeal process, and afterwards where an appeal is unsuccessful (see Chapter 10).

Illness

Children under 18 years who are ill either at home or in hospital are entitled to education in as far as can be accommodated with their illness. Hospitals may have a 'school' in the children's ward, and at the least there will be visiting peripatetic teachers from the local education authority who will assess and deliver appropriate education. Where young people are receiving treatment for mental health problems they are entitled to be involved in education provided this is not detrimental to their well-being. NICE guidance (2005) on depression states that inpatient facilities should be age appropriate and culturally enriching.

The phenomenon of fabricated and induced illness can lead to children missing school. Where a school or a practitioner is suspicious about school absence it is essential that joint working is instigated across all agencies, and that all records and information, including reports from private health care providers and alternative practitioners, concerning the child can be accessed or at least known about. The main issues here are safeguarding the physical or emotional health of the child, respecting the rights of the child, and preventing further abuse of the child through the health care system, either privately or through the NHS. The school nurse will need to liaise with adult health services to assess the parents' health and to put services into place for the family. The outcomes for these children can depend on the way this is handled and the extent to which the parents acknowledge the problem and work with agencies.

School nurses and others must be culturally aware of the practice of female circumcision (Female Genital Mutilation), which although illegal in this country may be accessed illegally here; alternatively, the child may be taken abroad for the abuse. Where there are concerns then the safeguarding guidelines should be followed.

Taking ill health in its widest sense, some children become school refusers through a variety of routes. This may be from bullying, by school staff as well as other pupils, or from anxiety related to achievement or performance, or from being diagnosed with a condition requiring medication such as asthma or diabetes, or from circumstances at home, such as parental illness, domestic abuse or a new baby, where they are concerned about what will happen when they are not at home. It may be that they have become a young carer without realising. The school, the educational welfare service and the school nurse will need to work together with the young person and their family to resolve the issues. This joint working, although ultimately more effective, is extremely time-consuming, and is an example of where 'time and motion' studies do not reflect the input of the nurse's, or any other worker's, time or the output in relation to the young person.

Teenage pregnancy

Britain has a well documented teenage pregnancy problem (Social Exclusion Unit, 1999; DfES, 2006) which has proved to need a long-term inter-agency response to reduce it. The 1999 report to the Social Exclusion unit identified sexual abuse in childhood, mental health problems, poverty, being in local authority care, youth offending and truancy as risk factors for teenage pregnancy. Practitioners, including midwives, involved with these young women must be sure to take these factors into account when booking and assessing their clients, and make sure that services are offered for the mother as well as for the pregnancy.

Teenage mothers often present late to ante-natal services, and so miss pre-conceptual and early ante-natal care. Often the young women were not intending pregnancy and continue with other behaviours, such as smoking, drinking alcohol or taking medicines or prescribed or illicit drugs, which have adverse effects on the pregnancy. Their babies on average have lower birth weights and higher infant mortality (ECM, 2007a). This reinforces the fact that public health nurses, such as school nurses, should be prioritising health promotion and sex and relationship education, including contraception to vulnerable young people (see Chapter 5). They should also be involved in strategic developments that ensure that services are meeting the needs of those with the poorest health outcomes.

Family Nurse Partnerships (ECM, 2008) have been piloted in some areas and provide intensive parenting support for vulnerable first-time mothers to promote breast feeding and other optimal health and well-being outcomes. Statistically, girls from areas of disadvantage are more likely to become pregnant (NRU, undated) and they may miss significant amounts of school. They may then not return to education or employment, with the consequence of poor employment opportunities leading to possible poverty, isolation and poor health outcomes. To break this cycle, it is essential that young people are supported to remain in education through pregnancy and afterwards to improve their own and their baby's life chances.

Health, social and education services have a responsibility to provide joined-up appropriate services which enable young teenage mothers to access education, and further education to facilitate this. Teenage mothers with prospects, it is hoped, will delay having a second child, and give a better start in life to the first child.

Homelessness

Many families are in temporary accommodation following domestic abuse, financial problems or environmental problems such as flooding (Shelter, 2006). Others are temporary residents, as they are asylum seekers, refugees or illegal immigrants. In all cases, the services are often geared towards the adults' agenda; children may not be able to attend their school as it is too far away, so they are out of school, bored and lonely. Temporary housing is often sub-standard and overcrowded, hygiene of communal kitchens and bathrooms may be poor and accidents are common. Community infections are readily contracted in such circumstances, but the family may not be registered with a local GP, and is unlikely to know how to access local services. Some areas employ 'homelessness' health visitors, who are often the first to realise that school-aged children have arrived at the refuge or temporary accommodation, and they alert education services and the school nurse.

NEETS

People under 18 years who are not in education, employment or training, are referred to as NEETS (ECM, 2007b). Across the UK, this accounts for about 10% of young people (Popam, 2003), though it is difficult to establish as they are a group often slipping into and out of education and employment. They are likely to have left school with few or no qualifications, and even where agencies encourage them to attend further education or 'on the job' training their attendance is poor. They do not identify that education and skills are a passport to financial stability and good health and social well-being. They will probably have significant other needs around issues of physical and mental health or family relationships, or they may have already come to the attention of the youth justice system (Prince's Trust, 2007).

There are higher numbers of NEETs in areas affected by deprivation and multi-generational unemployment and where neighbourhoods have become run down. Although there is some alternative employment, the young people have no family background which encourages them to develop different skills for a changing world. Without aspirations, these young people are at risk of becoming marginalised, leading to low incomes, depression, poor health and teenage pregnancy. Young people with learning difficulties, those leaving care, teenage mothers and young offenders are very likely to become NEETs.

Services

Children missing from education may never have started school, or they may have been withdrawn from school following a dispute, or have moved from the area but failed to enrol at another school, or they may leave primary school but never arrive at secondary school. It is the parents' responsibility to register them at a new school (Education Act, 1996). The police will be involved where children have run away, either from home or from care, and they will liaise with the education welfare service with any information about such children. If a young person cannot be persuaded to return home, or if they have been ejected from the family home, then counselling and mediation will be tried. If that fails then the young person may be offered temporary housing. This is variable, as those who are 16–18 years old, where there is pressure on supported housing, may well be housed in a hostel, where other itinerant adults live. This will expose them to the health risks of alcohol, smoking and drugs. They are unlikely to register with a GP or dentist, and they don't have the skills or facilities to be able to prepare and cook fresh nourishing food.

There are cases where unaccompanied children arrive in this country and are placed in the care of the local authority, but then disappear. In some cases the police find that this is connected to criminal activity involving child prostitution. Naturally, there are grave concerns for the health and well-being of such young people, but they themselves are often coerced into keeping quiet by perceived threats to their families at home. In all cases such as these, professionals will follow the local safeguarding guidelines.

All four countries in the United Kingdom have established mechanisms including monitoring and targeting in order to prevent children and young people from dropping out of school. However, there is no central list where details of a child's registered school are kept; each school maintains its own list, so they are not traced when they move to another area. Every statutory agency which deals with children is required, under Laming recommendations (2003), to record the school which the child attends. This information is, however, not checked, so unscrupulous parents can lie. Many education authorities organise regular 'truanting sweeps' with the local police and sometimes involving the local community, where school-aged children or their accompanying adult are asked to explain why the child is not in school that day. If applicable, the child is returned to school, or if unknown then this is followed up by the education welfare service.

Education welfare services work with parents and individual young people who have become alienated from school and will try to secure alternative education or work experience, in order to keep them within the statutory system. In cases where the child's behaviour has caused them to become excluded from school (this can happen as early as five years old), parenting programmes and contracts will be put in place to provide parents or carers with the skills they need to address the child's behaviour. New provisions under the Education and Inspections Act 2006 places a duty on parents to ensure that their excluded child is not found present in a public place during school hours, without a reasonable excuse, during the first five days of any exclusion. If found in such circumstances then the local authority or school can issue a penalty notice to the

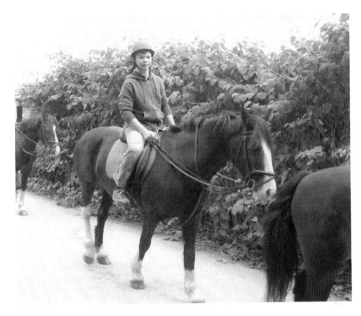

All children and young people spend a significant amount of their time outside the school setting.

parents. Failure to pay a fixed penalty notice could lead to a prosecution. Where parents desist or are unable to comply, the child may be taken into local authority care on the grounds of neglect (which may be unintentional) to ensure that his/her needs are met in order to access education which is his/her right.

In England, if a child is found to be not attending school, then the education authority will write to the parents demanding that they satisfy them within 15 days that the child is receiving suitable education (DfES, 2005). Failing that they will issue a 'school attendance order' to insist that the child attends a named school, and thereafter prosecute the parents for keeping the child from education, and ultimately take the child into local authority care.

Pupil referral units

There are some children and young people who because of illness, or exclusion from school, need to be educated outside of mainstream provision. They may be offered home tuition, though this is rare, or attendance at a 'pupil referral unit' These typically offer anger management, behaviour training and counselling individually and in small groups to enable pupils to return to mainstream school. Although entitled to full time education and a full curriculum, many of these young people either fail to attend full time, or have a reduced time table because of their difficulties, which means that they are out of school during the daytime and unsupervised. They are vulnerable to risk taking behaviour, and should be offered in depth sex and relationships education, and support around controlling or resisting alcohol, smoking and drugs. They may have missed significant amounts of school and lack basic knowledge about a healthy diet, the importance of good mental health, the dangers of substance misuse or the risk of catching sexually transmitted diseases, crucial to promoting their health and well-being . School nurses should prioritise these vulnerable children and regularly monitor their health status. They should work creatively and opportunistically within the multi-disciplinary team to enhance their emotional resilience, factual knowledge and confidence in choosing good health. Good record keeping is essential, as these young people may have missed out on immunisations, or may have diagnosed or undiagnosed illnesses for which they need regular medication or supervision. The school nurse will need to find any previous records and liaise with the client's GP.

It is recognised, however, that educational achievement and other outcomes varies widely, and the Children's Plan (DCSF, 2007b) has suggested experimenting with other forms of alternative provision, such as 'studio' schools with close links to business and vocational education, to try to re-engage those young people for whom academic qualifications are not seen as relevant.

The Connexions service was established in 2001 with a remit to provide a comprehensive support and guidance service to individual young people , particularly NEETS, through a dedicated personal adviser. Good quality information, advice and guidance regarding educational and vocational skills and training are necessary for young people, particularly where their parents may be unable to offer this. The Children's Plan (DCSF, 2007b) proposes that vulnerable young people such as care leavers will be entitled to a personal advisor up to the age of 25 if they want to continue in education.

Aiming High for Young People: a Ten Year Strategy for Positive Activities (HM Treasury, 2007) sets out a multi-agency approach to deal with those children and young people who need specific and sustained interventions in their lives if they are to fulfil their expectations. Education, health, social services, Connexions, drug and alcohol teams, the police and the voluntary sector must work together to deliver these additional outcomes, which will be monitored by Children's Trusts. Although emotional resilience and improved health are stated as desired outcomes, it is no coincidence that this is led by the Treasury, as the consequences of feckless and anarchic youths are expensive for the country. The targets are:

- Reduce the percentage of NEETS
- Increase participation in positive activities
- Reduce the proportion of young people using illegal drugs, alcohol or volatile substances

- Reduce under 18 conception rate
- Reduce the number of first-time entrants to the Criminal Justice System aged 10–17

The Welsh Assembly, in its document *The Learning Country: Vision into Action* (DELLS, 2007) has set a target to increase the percentage of young people in education, employment or training to 93% by 2010 through the youth gateway service. All countries' education systems try to identify pupils who are not achieving, in order to plan their 14–19 years pathway to prevent them from dropping out of education and the wider society.

The Scottish government has a NEET strategy and has established a NEET unit to monitor performance across agencies and identify gaps.

There are many small voluntary sector groups offering help to poor, vulnerable or disaffected children and young people, sometimes related to cultural or religious backgrounds, but more often from a neighbourhood perspective. Different charities are involved in schemes across the country to offer after-school and holiday care, respite care for young carers, and financial support to families and individuals. Where multi-agency working is the norm, statutory agencies are able to refer into these schemes, and practitioners should make it their duty to find out the remit of these groups and make sure of safeguarding issues before doing so.

Young offenders

The provision for young offenders across the country is extremely variable, and includes secure and community provision. Full assessment of the young person's mental, emotional, physical and educational needs is often lacking.

Barrett and Byford (2006) found that there were needs in mental health and social relationships, and that one in five had a learning disability. The fact that services may not be meeting these needs was not only to do with service providers. Many young people declined to engage with services offered, particularly those in community settings. There were concurrent problems of alcohol and drug use. Secure accommodation may give access to education, but engagement and continuity are a challenge. Targeted multi-agency work at neighbourhood level has been instigated to try to turn young people away from drifting into crime through boredom. Positive Futures is a social inclusion programme, aimed at 10–19 year olds, based on sports and leisure activities. It aims to use sport to engage young people to make decisions for themselves and to take up education and employment.

Conclusion

Children and young people who are out of school and education do not constitute a homogeneous group; there are a variety of different reasons. Many, perhaps the majority, have severely compromised futures. They may not value academic education, as they cannot succeed, and their family backgrounds do not support it. In many cases they have problems which affect them today, and which lay down further problems for the future, but their families have limited resources to help them. This may be compounded by poor mental and emotional health, learning disability, drug and alcohol use, relationship problems, poverty and a deprived social environment. Sensible planning for the future, aspiring to succeed or 'choosing health' in this context, is an unrealistic expectation. The problems which these children and young people face are outside of their sphere of influence, and that of their families. Promotion of their health and well-being involves health, education, social care, the police and the legal system. Indeed, it needs to be addressed by society as a whole.

References

Barrett, B. and Byford, S. (2006) Mental health provision for young offenders: service use and cost. *Journal of Psychiatry* **188**, 541–6.

Community Care and Health (Scotland) Act (2002) http://www.opsi.gov.uk/legislation/scotland/acts2002/asp_20020005_en_1/; accessed 20 February 2008.

Dearden, C. and Becker, S. (1998) *Young Carers in the United Kingdom: A Profile.* Carers National Association, London.

Dearden, C. and Becker, S. (2004) *Young Carers in the UK: the 2004 Report.* Carers UK, London.

Department for Children, Schools and Families (2007a) Guidance *on the Education (School Attendance Targets) (England) Regulations.* http://www.dfes.gov.uk/schoolattendance/attendancetargets/index.cfm; accessed 20 February 2008.

Department for Children, Schools and Families (2007b) *The Children's Plan: Building Brighter Futures.* Stationery Office, Norwich.

Department for Education and Skills (2004) *Every Child Matters.* Stationery Office, London.

Department for Education and Skills (2005) *Is Your Child Missing Out? School Attendance Information for Parents.* DfES, Nottingham.

Department of Education (Northern Ireland) (2007) *Non Attendance.* http://www.deni.gov.uk/; accessed 17 February 2008.

Department for Education and Skills (2006) *Teenage Pregnancy Next Steps: Guidance for Local Authorities and Primary Care Trusts on Effective Delivery of Local Strategies.* DfES Publications, Nottingham.

Department for Education, Lifelong Learning and Skills (2007) *The Learning Country: Vision onto Action*. Welsh Assembly Government, Cardiff.

Department for Education and Skills (DfES) (1996) *The Education Act*. DfES, London.

Every Child Matters (2007a) *About the Teenage Pregnancy Strategy*. http://www.everychildmatters.gov.uk/health/teenagepregnancy/about/; accessed 20 February 2008.

Every Child Matters (2007b) *Young People Not in Education, Employment or Training*. http://www.everychildmatters.gov.uk/ete/neet/; accessed 16 February 2008.

Every Child Matters (2008) *Health-led Parenting Support*. http://www.everychildmatters.gov.uk/parents/healthledsupport/; accessed 20 February 2008.

HM Government/Department for Children, Schools and Families (2007) *Aiming High for Young People: a Ten Year Strategy for Positive Activities*. HM Government/ Department for Children, Schools and Families, London.

Hopwood, V., O'Neill, L., Castro, G. and Hodgson, B. (2007) *The Prevalence of Home Education in England (2006)*. http://www.dfes.gov.uk/research/data/uploadfiles/ RB827.pdf; accessed 20 February 2008.

Laming, Lord (2003) *The Victoria Climbié Inquiry: Report of an Inquiry by Lord Laming*. Stationery Office, London.

MORI (2004) *MORI Youth Survey 2004*. Youth Justice Board for England and Wales. http://www.yjb.gov.uk/Publications/Scripts/prodView.asp?idproduct=187&eP; accessed 20 February 2008.

Neighbourhood Renewal Unit (Undated) *Health Teenage Pregnancy*. http://www.neighbourhood.gov.uk/page.asp?id=725; accessed 20 February 2008.

National Institute for Health and Clinical Excellence (2005) *Depression in Young People*. http://www.nice.org.uk/guidance/CG28/; accessed 20 February 2008.

Ofsted (2004) *Out of School: a Survey of the Educational Support and Provision for Pupils Not in School*. Stationery Office, London.

Popham, I. (2003) *Research on Actions and Other Factors That Can Contribute to a Reduction in the Numbers of Young People Not in Education, Employment or Training* [NEET]. Connexions. http://www.connexions.gov.uk/partnerships/publications/connexpubs/index.cfm?Fuseaction=DocumentDetails&DocumentID=39 2; accessed 20 February 2008.

Prince's Trust (2007) *The Cost of Exclusion; Counting the Cost of Youth Disadvantage in the UK*. Prince's Trust, London.

Scottish Government News (2007) *Attendance and Absence in Scottish Schools 2006/07*. http://www.scottishexecutive.gov.uk/News/Releases/2007/12/12095057 /; accessed 20 February 2008.

Shelter (2006) *What is Homelessness?* http://england.shelter.org.uk/advice/advice-498.cfm#wipLive-7073-3; accessed 12 February 2008.

Social Exclusion Unit (1999) *Teenage Pregnancy*. Stationery Office, London.

Trades Union Congress (2001) *One in Ten School Kids Play Truant to Work*. http://www.tuc.org.uk/em_research/tuc-2973-f0.cfm; accessed 20 February 2008.

UN Millennium Development Goals (2000) http://www.un.org/millenniumgoals/; accessed 20 February 2008.

CHAPTER 13

Working together to promote the health of school age children

Jane Wright

Key themes

- Collaborative working within the education, health and social sectors to promote the health of school age children
- Examples of good practice: what works, what are the barriers?

Introduction: the context of change

This chapter will explore some of the current thinking around working together to promote the health and well-being of school age children and young people. Concepts of developing partnerships for change will be explored as demands for restructuring continue, and the perceived barriers to working together will be discussed. There has been a persistent emphasis on promoting the health and well-being of individuals and populations over the decades since the World Health Organization (WHO) declaration of 'health for all by 2000', in 1978 (WHO, 1978). Primary care was identified as a top priority across the world with emphasis on bringing health services as close as possible to where people live and work. The attainment of optimum health as a world-wide social goal included the concepts of collaboration, including 'suitably trained' professionals working together in teams (WHO, 1978). The right of individuals to participate in the planning and implementation of their health care was also identified within the declaration. There have been subsequent global conferences to review progress worldwide and although definitions of health have changed, the fundamental concepts of building alliances across different sectors to promote health; assessing need, and recognising the right of individuals to participate in decision making, remain the same (WHO, 2005). There has also been a continued drive to make health promotion a core responsibility of all governments across the world because health is seen as a major determinant of socio-economic and political development (WHO, 2005). Therefore, it is in a country's best interest to ensure the health of its population and it can also be argued that promoting health cannot be confined to the health services alone (Law, 2003).

Since 1978 in the UK, the fundamental concepts of health promotion from the WHO declaration have been reproduced within government policy documents by successive governments (see Figure 13.1). The Children's Plan 2007 reflected the concepts of listening to children, young people and parents and designing services locally, around identified need (Department for Children, Schools and Families [DCSF], 2007). It also acknowledged the need to examine the way professionals and groups work together and consider changes in practice to meet need.

The threats to the health of children and young people have changed dramatically over the last hundred years. They now include obesity and other eating disorders, smoking, mental health problems, sexual health, drugs and alcohol, and these are discussed in other chapters. There are also continuing health inequalities and more children and young people living with long-term conditions into adulthood. Health and social care services have been required to re-think models of service delivery to address these changing needs and there is a consequent growing burden of costs. Both the NHS Plan (DH, 2000a) and the Wanless Review (Wanless, 2002) recommended increases in staff in the NHS to address these needs which, according to Wanless (2007), has been achieved, but this increase is not necessarily in the areas which can contribute to improving the health of children and families such as in School Nursing, Health Visiting, Community Children's Nursing and Learning Disability Nursing.

Budgets for these areas are often cut in favour of other services, and while this continues to happen, progress in addressing the determinants of health, and consequently, outcomes for children in the greatest need may be limited (Wanless, 2007). One of the recognised difficulties is that health promotion activity has remained hard to measure effectively, as no official figures have been available (Wanless, 2007). There are examples of good practice, but the evidence that particular models work, particularly in the long term, is patchy, with a lack of evaluation activity as a key problem (Whitehead, 2003). We can make intelligent assumptions that if we prevent a child from becoming obese, smoking, drinking, taking drugs or taking risks we will save money in the future (Audit Commission, 2007), but unless there is evidence, then the resources to support these interventions may not continue. This has been recognised worldwide with calls from WHO in Mexico (2000) and Bangkok

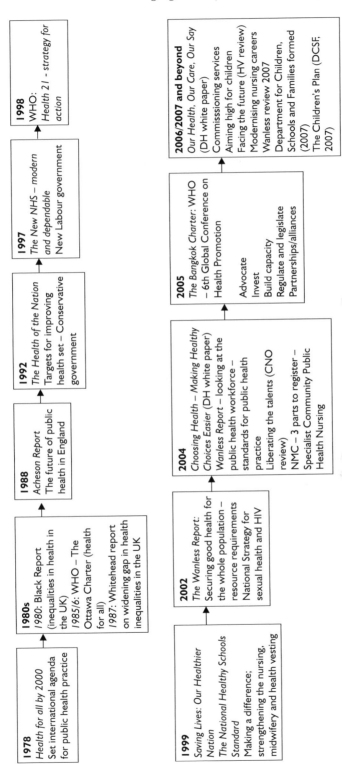

Figure 13.1 Time line since 1978: overview of public health policy.

(2005) to strengthen the evidence base for health promotion in all countries (WHO, 2000, 2005). Wanless (2004) also suggested that more investment was required to develop expertise in the areas of research techniques to demonstrate the need for resources. Clinical effectiveness or audit departments within Trusts have grown with support from the Audit Commission, which is an independent organisation monitoring the efficiency of public services. The Audit Commission has a responsibility to ensure that local strategic partnerships are taking the necessary steps to improve health and well-being in the local community (Audit Commission, 2007). The Audit Commission works in partnership with the National Audit Office, the Healthcare Commission, and the Commission for Social Care and Inspection and in 2008/2009, children's health and well-being as well as the funding for children's services was part of the Health Studies Consultation (Audit Commission, 2007). All these bodies are government organisations concerned with the quality and consistency of health and social care.

Given these ongoing difficulties in promoting the health of children and young people with a limited workforce, the issue of working in partnerships becomes more crucial. A close look at the current training of public health, health and social care staff and a consideration of the changes required to ensure quality care, including preventative services is needed. There are common themes in all these areas in terms of standards for practice, which include collaborative working, working with and for communities, leadership and management and research and development (Public Health Register, 2001; Nursing and Midwifery Council [NMC], 2004)

There has been a drive towards interprofessional learning and education, with the logical argument that learning together will improve understanding of roles and responsibilities, support collaborative working and improve quality of care and services (Creating an Interprofessional Workforce [CIPW], 2006). The aim of CIPW was to produce a learning framework to support collaborative practice and partnership working in health and social care as a response to recommendations from policy documents. The review found that the success of interprofessional learning and development varied widely across the country and recommended that there should be a nationally coordinated approach; this is an ongoing project.

There is also emphasis on working with clients to provide services according to their needs which involves forming partnerships and consulting service users. It is interesting to note, however, that the Children's Workforce Development Council (CWDC) highlighted that children and young people felt that they were sometimes 'over-consulted', with little happening as a result of the information gained (CWDC, 2007). This demonstrates that consultations must produce action, otherwise the consultation process remains a token gesture. There is an attempt to move away from a victim-blaming culture towards one which supports and respects individual decision-making processes but which ensures that families have real choices to make in the first place. These strategies include the social marketing principles of considering the patient as the client, but they also include a drive towards entrepreneurial activity from providers of services (Health Development Agency [HDA], 2003; National Social Marketing [NSM], 2006). Health may be considered to be one of a nation's assets as it is shown that good levels of health are associated with overall well-being leading to better productivity (Nuffield Council on Bioethics, 2007). If another key asset of a nation are its children and young people it makes sense to promote their health to ensure a future productive and economically stable society. The question is how this can be effectively achieved.

Overview of children's services development: reality and rhetoric

In terms of promoting the health of children and young people, there have been particular policy drivers for a more concerted effort to form effective partnerships (DH, 2004a; DfES, 2005) (see Figure 13.2). There is also a continued drive towards more emphasis on primary care, and moving services and training into the community (DH, 2006b).

The overall intention of government strategy across departments has been to bring services together around the needs of children, young people and families with a more flexible model of service delivery in order to improve outcomes for children. The priority in the first instance must be to safeguard vulnerable children and young people and, as previous reports have shown, this requires cross-sector working, communication and cooperation (Kennedy, 2001; Laming, 2003). The Kennedy report on paediatric cardiac surgery at Bristol Royal Infirmary highlighted the need for specifically trained staff to work with children and recognised the need for groups and individuals to acknowledge the contribution of others in the service of patients (Kennedy, 2001). *The Options for Excellence Review* (DH/DfES, 2006a) discussed the future of social care in the UK in the light of *Every Child Matters* (ECM) (DH/DfES, 2004a) and *Our Health. Our Care. Our Say* (DH, 2006a). It also outlined the need for new ways of working and highlighted areas of good practice where health, education and social care had come together to provide a high-quality service. It recognised common skills that are required when working with children and acknowledged the consultation between the Nursing and Midwifery Council (NMC), the General Social Care Council (GSCC), and the General Teaching Council (GTC) which produced an interprofessional values statement following the *Every Child Matters* White Paper (NMC/GSCC/GTC, 2004; DH/DfES, 2004a). The values statement outlined the key attributes required for all prac-

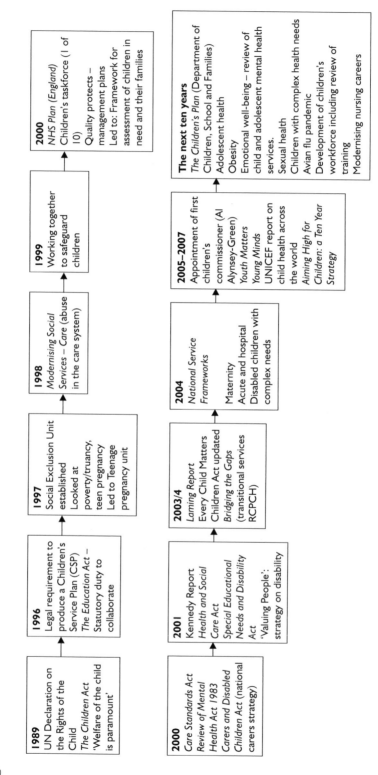

1989
UN Declaration on the Rights of the Child
The Children Act – 'Welfare of the child is paramount'

1996
Legal requirement to produce a Children's Service Plan (CSP)
The Education Act – Statutory duty to collaborate

1997
Social Exclusion Unit established
Looked at poverty/truancy, teen pregnancy
Led to Teenage pregnancy unit

1998
Modernising Social Services – Care (abuse in the care system)

1999
Working together to safeguard children

2000
NHS Plan (England)
Children's taskforce (1 of 10)
Quality protects – management plans
Led to: Framework for assessment of children in need and their families

2000
Care Standards Act
Review of Mental Health Act 1983
Carers and Disabled Children Act (national carers strategy)

2001
Kennedy Report
Health and Social Care Act
Special Educational Needs and Disability Act
'*Valuing People*': strategy on disability

2003/4
Laming Report
Every Child Matters
Children Act updated
Bridging the Gaps (transitional services RCPCH)

2004
National Service Frameworks
Maternity
Acute and hospital
Disabled children with complex needs

2005–2007
Appointment of first children's commissioner (Al Alynsey-Green)
Youth Matters
Young Minds
UNICEF report on child health across the world
Aiming High for Children: a Ten Year Strategy

The next ten years
The Children's Plan (Department of Children, School and Families)
Adolescent health
Obesity
Emotional well-being – review of child and adolescent mental health services.
Sexual health
Children with complex health needs
Avian flu pandemic
Development of children's workforce including review of training
Modernising nursing careers

Figure 13.2 Time line since 1989: Overview of health and social policy affecting children's services.

titioners working with children and young people and was developed with the *Common Core of Skills and Knowledge for the Children's Workforce* guidance produced in 2005 (HM Government, 2005). The partners who developed this guidance include Skills for Health, the Children's Workforce Development Council, the GSCC and voluntary agencies such as the NSPCC. These partners were looking to service managers to develop inter-agency training and establish greater shared language and understanding across different sectors and it is hoped that it may be used as a tool for workforce planning (HM Government, 2005).

There is often a clear gap between what government policy is outlining for practice and the reality. Resource issues in the community and primary care have continued to make it extremely difficult to achieve health for all children in all circumstances. The government is committed to decentralisation and devolving responsibility locally and this has meant a move towards a commissioning structure with PCTs (DH, 2004a). PCTs have become responsible for commissioning services to meet need but, when a financial restriction is imposed, there has to be prioritisation, and health promoting services, staff training and continuing professional education are often the ones cut (Wanless, 2007; CIPW, 2007). This makes it extremely difficult to achieve major change and creates a demoralised workforce, which is not conducive to innovation and creative practice. Without development of the local workforce (including their professional development), improvements in leadership and management and a look at recruitment and retention, achievement of targets will be impossible (DH/DfES, 2006a; Wanless, 2007).

There also continues to be disparity between areas where there are examples of good practice but in others there has been little development (DCSF, 2007). This is supported by statistics which indicates that there continues to be health inequality, social exclusion and poverty in the UK, demonstrated by research from the Joseph Rowntree Foundation (Palmer *et al.*, 2005). Although this is acknowledged by policy makers, resources are, in some areas, not matching need, and this has been highlighted in the *Children's Plan: Building Brighter Futures* (DCSF, 2007).

The concepts of assessing need and targeting resources are explicit in government policy and the establishment of Children's Trusts is a step towards refining service to meet the specific needs of children and young people. The development of Children's Trusts has been an example of working together to provide services for children in a coordinated way and they have been discussed in other chapters. However, their relevance to working in partnership needs exploration. The theoretical base for introducing Children's Trusts would appear sound as they provide an opportunity to bring professionals together under one management structure. This allows managers to plan training for staff more effectively, listen to young people and their families and tailor services to individual and community need. Children's centres in some

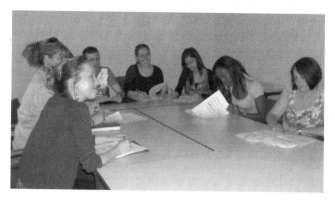

Working in partnership promotes health and well-being.

areas provided opportunities for staff to be physically together as well as theoretically, which also makes logical sense and encourages better understanding, communication and collaboration.

There were 35 Children's Trust pathfinders across England, and in March 2007 the three-year review which evaluated the effectiveness of the model was published (University of East Anglia [UEA] National Children's Bureau [NCB], 2007). The 35 pathfinders accounted for 20% of children and young people aged 0–19 in England and were spread throughout the country. The positive aspects of the review were that they have provided a platform for changing the service provision for children and young people. The review demonstrated that it is possible for local authorities, health services, police and other relevant agencies to work together to plan children's services, but the process of change is often very slow. The pathfinder Trusts worked in different ways to fund services; some pooled budgets from different agencies through legal agreements and others aligned budgets and shared information on spending. Legal agreements were essential to protect or 'ring fence' money, particularly for the health sector to prevent money being redirected into other areas. The Audit Commission examined these financial issues in 2008/2009, in particular looking at pooling monies as a more efficient way of using the budgets (Audit Commission, 2007).

The barriers have also included the complexities of managing change across different agencies and engaging different professionals in the process (e.g. Head Teachers and General Practitioners). The difficulties included structural and cultural differences between different agencies for example, different accountability frameworks, use of language and understanding of others roles. These barriers across professional boundaries and cultures have also been highlighted in other reviews of practice, collaborative working and learning together (Audit Commission, 2007; CIPW, 2007). It has remained too early to provide concrete evidence of the contribution to the five outcomes for children and young people outlined in *Every Child Matters* (DH/DfES, 2004a) but, according to the review, 25 sites reported specific examples of improvements and some have also highlighted an improvement in the efficiency of service provision.

Extended schools can also offer opportunities for partnership working and are discussed in Chapter 2. In terms of working together, they provide further opportunities for agencies to come together to plan, implement and evaluate appropriate services. Extended schools may also allow the further development of health services for young people such as sexual and emotional health services. School Nurses (SNs) have developed drop-ins in their schools for some time across the country and in some areas these have been multi-agency. The school nurse development pack (DH/DfES, 2006b) and the NMC *Standards of Proficiency for Specialist Community Public Health Nursing* (NMC, 2004) have outlined competencies in collaborative working as part of public health practice. School nurses are ideally placed for collaboration as they work with a range of professionals across many sectors: Connexions workers, social care staff, voluntary agencies, mental health workers, community leaders, parents, carers, children and young people and education (DH/DfES, 2006b). Their training includes developing the communication skills required to negotiate with schools, assess need and lead projects according to that need (NMC, 2004). Negotiation skills were highlighted in the review of Children's Trusts (UEA/NCB 2007) as a key to successful partnership working.

School nurses have also developed their skills as providers of advice and care and also as gatekeepers, guiding young people towards appropriate professional help if necessary. *Aiming High for Young People: A Ten Year Strategy for Positive Activities* (DH, 2007) looks to develop this multi-agency working further in order that young people can access help from a range of professionals more easily and to give young people more choice in their access to services. Where multi-agency services have already been set up successfully close to where young people are, the evidence suggests that young people are more likely to access the service and therefore achieve the outcomes from *Every Child Matters* (DH/DfES, 2004a). The evidence from a range of sources also suggests that talking to young people about the most appropriate services for them may be more effective than a top-down approach, imposing services that adults think they need (HM Government, 2005; CWDC, 2007). The philosophy in health and social care has developed in this direction, where users are consulted about their care, both nationally as in *Our Health, Our Care, Our Say* (DH, 2006a) and locally with patient liaison groups and open meetings in primary care (UEA/NCM, 2007). Effective communication with children and young people is also explicit in the *Common Core of Skills and Knowledge for the Children's Workforce* (HM Government, 2005).

The key to successful services for young people in schools also hinges on the cooperation of the school, governors and parents and this can be difficult, particularly around sexual health services. However, given the success of some projects and the lack of widespread public outcry, more schools are considering their pastoral care and developing services in schools across the country. Extended schools may help this process by encouraging schools to engage in the broader aspects of life and, in particular, the health and well-being of children and young people. It will also make it more acceptable for young people to stay on after school hours without being questioned, giving them opportunities to access services.

There is recognition that the health problems affecting the population start in childhood with the new public health threats of obesity, smoking, poor emotional health and physical activity (Wanless, 2007). To address these, as well as the problems of the rise in teenage pregnancy and sexually transmitted infections (STIs) will undoubtedly require a broad approach using both top-down and bottom-up strategies. A multi-system approach is the most likely to succeed as this will address the different needs that young people have, their diverse learning styles and their individual circumstances.

Models for delivery

The 6th global conference on health promotion in Bangkok (WHO, 2005) provided a framework for promoting child health both globally and domestically. The key elements for successful child health promotion can be outlined as advocacy for health (safeguarding), investment in policy and resources, building partnerships and alliances across all sectors and developing research to support sustainable projects (see Table 13.1).

The National Service Framework for Children, Young People and Maternity Services (DH/DfES, 2004b) developed a framework for child health promotion which built on the global framework outlined in Mexico in 2000 (WHO, 2000).

Table 13.1 The Bangkok Charter (WHO, 2005).

- **Advocate** for health based on human rights and solidarity
- **Invest** in sustainable policies, actions and infrastructure to address the determinants of health
- **Build capacity** for policy development, leadership, health promotion practice, knowledge transfer and research, and health literacy
- **Regulate and legislate** to ensure a high level of protection from harm and enable equal opportunity for health and well-being for all people
- **Partner and build alliances** with public, private, nongovernmental and international organizations and civil society to create sustainable actions.

This included building on the concepts of working in partnerships with other agencies and also with individuals, families and communities. This is supportive of the overall aims of health promotion strategy to enable people to achieve control over their own health through collective action (Webster and French, 2003; WHO, 2005). This collective action should be firstly at a strategic level, where different agencies are required to plan, implement and evaluate services together. Secondly, action should be operational, where policy is implemented and thirdly, individual action at the grass roots of the service itself (Day, 2006). For example, there may be a strategic plan locally to reduce teenage pregnancy which is implemented operationally by managers of the school nursing teams and then individually in the schools by the SNs by setting up multi-agency sexual health services. The most successful local projects may be those that are initiated at the grass roots levels by practitioners who are passionate about a particular topic or become motivated by frustration at a gap in services.

Building partnerships

Change is an inevitable fact of life, but those working in the NHS over the last decade, particularly in primary care, have seen unprecedented change and restructuring which has often left staff feeling demotivated to tackle anything new (DH, 2004a). Those working with children and young people have had to deal with both positive and negative implications of government policy. Government rhetoric is positive about a sustained effort to put children at the forefront of reform: for example the appointment of a children's commissioner and a government minister for children and families. However, in 2007, there continued to be depressing news about children living in poverty, increasing youth crime and a UNICEF report that the UK featured towards the bottom of a survey about the quality of life for children and young people in Europe (UNICEF Innocenti Research Centre, 2007).

WHO uses the terms 'collaboration', 'building healthy alliances' and 'working in teams' when discussing health promotion activity (WHO, 2005). Healthy alliances can be defined as building partnerships for improving health which can be collective action where there is an attempt to improve the social and environmental factors which impact on individual health (Scriven, 1998). It can also be individual partnerships, for example on a one to one basis with a young person or a relationship with a family. This suggests that working together can be with a wide range of individuals and groups, not necessarily professionals or statutory agencies. The term 'partnership' may be a useful one as it implies a 'sharing' of information, responsibility or workload. The term also suggests a contractual agreement which could be either formal or infor-

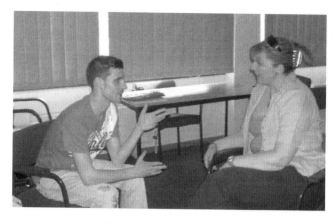

Engaging young people effectively is vital for successful health promotion.

mal. A formal agreement or partnership needs to be formed within a Children's Trust for example, but a meeting with a parent or young person may be more informal. However, outcomes from the arrangement still need to be agreed in any situation for positive action to occur.

The behaviour of children and young people has become a concern for society in recent years, with a rise in youth crime, antisocial behaviour and a perceived lack of discipline in schools, the home and the community. Ashton (2000) described this increasing fragmentation of society and communities in relation to public health, with the premise that health and social problems are closely linked. He suggested that some of the causes were poor leadership, a lack of a shared ethical framework or common values and a sense of powerlessness. Speaking in 2000, Ashton also described Arnstein's ladder of participation, which places partnership towards the top of the ladder where there is a degree of power achieved by the citizen (Ashton, 2000). This has developed in the form of community participation with an emphasis on effective consultations. The government has explored the possibility of forming contracts or partnerships with parents, young people, the community and schools to improve overall behaviour and outcomes for children (Home Office, 2006; DH, 2007; DCSF, 2007). This of course, must be part of broader, collective action by society as a whole to improve the conditions in which people live, learn and work. The concepts of creating supportive environments, building social capital and introducing citizenship in schools all rely on developing a common goal through successful partnerships or alliances (Scriven, 1998; Costello and Haggart 2003).

This will depend upon issues such as trust, respect, effective communication and negotiation skills. Clear and effective leadership will enable sustainable change to occur and this may depend on a leader's ability to develop shared commitment to the process with common, agreed goals clearly identified. This clarity of purpose is important to ensure that if the leader leaves a project, it remains sustainable. Leadership and management have become an integral part of health and social care courses and are explicit within public health standards for training (Public Health Register, 2001; NMC, 2004).

Social marketing: what is it and how does it encourage partnerships?

As well as tackling the broader determinants of health such as poverty and inequality, individual lifestyle and consideration of behavioural change remains a part of health promotion strategy. There must be recognition that there is a balance between what a government can do and what individuals and their families can do to achieve optimum health (Norton, 1998).

The National Social Marketing Centre was commissioned by government as part of *Choosing Health* (DH, 2004b) to develop the concepts of social marketing as a way of promoting health. The principles of social marketing include placing people at the centre of policy making and developing effective partnerships nationally, locally and with individuals. There is also the recommendation to stop what is not working and re-think action (National Social Marketing Centre [NSM], 2006). This supports the view that any initiative needs to produce evidence of successful outcomes and this will require staff to improve their skills of research to demonstrate effectiveness (Wanless, 2004). It is clear that simply providing young people with information about their health is not enough to encourage them to make positive choices. There are many other factors that compete for a young person's attention while they are growing up and the power of seeking pleasurable activity is great. The consideration of incentives for making healthier choices and offering alternatives may be a way forward; for example, exchanging unhealthy pleasurable experiences for more healthy ones. While this may be viewed as persuasive or manipulative health promotion strategy (Norton 1998), it can also be argued that this approach may be more likely to work with young people.

With the consumer or client at the centre, social marketing is about considering all aspects of behaviour and what affects behaviour change and how that can be influenced. The aim is to consider the person (young person in this case) in the context of their individual lives and where they are starting from and particularly developing services around those needs rather than a person fitting into the services that are available. In terms of social marketing, this is developing insight into why young people behave in certain ways and what influences their behaviour at different stages of their lives. An understanding of human development and behavioural theories is becoming a part of courses offering training in the skills and knowledge to work with children and young people (HM Government, 2005). It is particularly important to consider influences on behaviour at different stages in development to improve communication and develop appropriate services. The environment will have a huge impact on their behaviour: transitions in their lives such as changing school, change of peer groups, family dynamics and financial circumstances will all impact on behavioural choices. Risk-taking, self-harming behaviour and problems with mental health have been identified as issues for further research and development and increasing understanding of these issues is very important for all those working in education, health and social care and improvements will depend on working together (DCSF, 2007).

It is also important to continue the drive towards bringing services to where people are, and in relation to young people, this is often in the virtual world of the computer. While there continue to be understandable concerns about the use of Internet sites, they can be used effectively as part of a wider approach to supporting young people at specific developmental stages. Technology, such as mobile phones and internet social networks, has enabled young people to seek help anonymously. For example, in some areas, school nurses have used text messaging services to give support and advice to young people. *Aiming High for Young People: a Ten Year Strategy for Positive Activities* (DH, 2007) introduced 'teen life checks', online to enable young people to access information about their health and health services anonymously from a reliable source (Teen Life Checks, 2008). This requires an understanding of young people, their development and how effective communication can be established, and these, among other specialised skills, are required by all those working with children and young people (HM Government, 2005).

The most successful projects in schools are those that include a 'whole school' approach involving, and keeping informed, all members of staff and effecting a cultural change within the school environment, and possibly attitudes towards health and well-being (Licence, 2004; DfES, 2004). There is recognition that attainment in education will promote better outcomes later in life (DH, 2007). It is also acknowledged that schools should be healthy environments for this attainment to be achieved (DfEE, 2003; DfES, 2004). One problem is that working with schools is difficult when there are so many demands from other areas, such as national league tables, statutory testing of children and no standard requirement for concerted personal, health and social education (PHSE). Schools are complex environments, and research in schools, particularly from outside agencies, about the most appropriate health promotion initiatives may be problematic given these restraints on time. Once there is recognition by schools that improved health for pupils will ensure a better environment for learning, and consequent overall achievements, there is more chance of successful projects. The Healthy Schools Initiative (DfEE, 2003; DfES, 2004) has been an example of this where, although slow to start, schools are now recognising the benefits of a healthy environment and are becoming engaged with 90% of schools joining the scheme and 53% achieving Healthy Schools Status (Healthy Schools, 2008).

Conclusion

This chapter has raised issues around current policy for children's services in the UK. There is a historical background to health promotion which supports the current drive to build children's services around where they live and what they need rather than fitting them into already existing services. This seems a very positive and worthwhile agenda with good opportunities to make a difference to children's and young people's lives. There are difficulties with resources for health promotion activities, and without forward planning around the future workforce and appropriate training in the right areas this agenda may not be achieved. The skills and knowledge required to promote the health of school-age children are outlined in the *Common Core Skills for the Children's Work-force* and they include the ability to work in partnership for a common goal, the knowledge to provide evidence to support initiatives, and the skill to lead and manage sustainable projects to improve outcomes for children and young people. This will require a commitment to drive forward the children's agenda from the ground as well as the political will from above. It will require new ways of working with a range of groups and individuals and there are already good examples of this in the establishment of Children's Trusts. There is also a commitment to address some of the difficulties of professionals working across boundaries and inter-professional learning and training is continuing to be a developing priority. With all these changes, there are good opportunities for practitioners to make a real difference to the outcomes for children and young people.

References

Ashton, J. R. (2000) *Governance, Health and the new Citizenship*. Inaugural lecture at Liverpool John Moores University. http://www.nwpho.org.uk/lectures/ja04062001. pdf; accessed 20 January 2008.

Audit Commission (2007) *Health Studies Consultation*. Audit Commission, London.

Children's Workforce Development Council (2007) *Building the Vision: Developing and Implementing the Local Integrated Children's Workforce Strategies*. CWDC, Leeds.

Creating an Interprofessional Workforce (2007) *Report of the CIPW working group.* CIPW/DH, London.

Costello, J. and Haggart, M. (2003) *Public Health and Society.* Palgrave Macmillan, Basingstoke.

Day, J. (2006) *Interprofessional Working.* Nelson Thornes, Cheltenham.

Department for Education and Employment (DfEE) (2003) *National Healthy School Standard.* DfEE, Nottingham.

Department for Children, Schools and Families (2007) *The Children's Plan.* DCSF, London.

Department for Education and Skills (2004) *Healthy Living Blueprint for Schools.* DfES, Nottingham.

Department for Education and Skills (2005) *Children's Workforce Strategy: a Strategy to Build a World-class Workforce for Children and Young People.* DfES, London.

Department of Health/Department for Education and Skills (2004a) *Every Child Matters.* DfES, London.

Department of Health/Department for Education and Skills (2004b) *National Service Framework for Children, Young People and Maternity Services: Executive Summary.* DH, London.

Department of Health/Department for Education and Skills (2006a) *Options For Excellence: Building the Social Care Workforce of the Future.* DH, London.

Department of Health/Department for Education and Skills (2006b) *School Nurse: Practice Development Resource Pack.* DH, London.

Department of Health (2000a) *The NHS Plan.* DH, London.

Department of Health (2004a) *Practice-Based Commissioning: Promoting Clinical Engagement.* DH, London.

Department of Health (2004b) *Choosing Health: Making Healthy Choices Easier.* DH, London

Department of Health (2006a) *Our Health, Our Care, Our Say* DH, London.

Department of Health (2006b) *Modernising Nursing Careers.* DH London.

Department of Health (2007) *Aiming High for Young People: a Ten Year Strategy for Positive Activities.* DH, London.

Health Development Agency (2003) *Supporting PCT Nurse Leads in Working with Complexity; Leading with Emergence, Innovation and Adaptation.* HDA, London.

Healthy Schools (2008) National Healthy Schools Programme Progress Report. http://www.everychildmatters.gov.uk/health/healthyschools/; accessed 20 January 2008.

HM Government (2005) *Common Core of Skills and Knowledge for the Children's Workforce.* DfES, London.

Home Office (2006) *Respect Action Plan.* Home Office, London.

Kennedy, I. (2001) *Learning from Bristol: the Report of the Public Inquiry Into Children's Heart Surgery At the Bristol Royal Infirmary 1984–1995.* The Bristol Royal Infirmary Inquiry, Bristol.

Laming, Lord (2003) *The Victoria Climbié Inquiry: Report of an Inquiry by Lord Laming.* Stationery Office, London.

Law, C. (2003) Policy for Child Health in the United Kingdom. *Pediatrics,* **112**(3), 722–4

Licence, K. (2004) Promoting and protecting the health of children and young people. *Child Care: Health and Development*, **30**(6), 623–35.

National Social Marketing (2006) *It's Our Health*. National Social Marketing Centre, London. http://www.nsms.org.uk/images/CoreFiles/NCCSUMMARYItsOurHealthJune2006.pdf; accessed 10 December 2007.

NMC, GSCC, GTC (2004) *Working Together for a Better Future*. http://www.nmc-uk.org/aArticle.aspx?ArticleID=2344; accessed 11 January 2008.

Norton L (1998) Health promotion and health education: what role should the nurse adopt in practice? *Journal of Advanced Nursing*, **28**(6), 1269–75.

Nuffield Council on Bioethics (2007) *Public Health: Ethical Issues*. Nuffield Council on Bioethics, London.

Nursing and Midwifery Council (2004) *Standards of Proficiency for Specialist Commuity Public Health Nurses*. NMC, London.

Palmer, G., Carr, J. and Kenway, P. (2005) *Monitoring Poverty and Social Exclusion in the UK 2005*. Joseph Rountree Foundation. London.

Public Health Register (2001) *National Standards for Specialist Practice in Public Health*. Healthwork UK, London.

Scriven, A. (1998) *Alliances in Health Promotion: Theory and Practice*. Macmillan, London.

Teen Life Checks (2008) *Teen Life Checks: Check it Before You Wreck It*. http://www.teenlifecheck.co.uk/; accessed 20 January 2008.

UNICEF Innocenti Research Centre (2007). *Child Poverty in Perspective: an Overview of Child Well-being in Rich Countries*. Innocenti Research Centre, Florence.

University of East Anglia/National Children's Bureau (2007) *Children's Trusts Pathfinders: Innovative Partnerships for Improving the Well-being of Children and Young People. National Evaluation of Children's Trusts Pathfinders*. UEA/NCB, Norwich. http://www.everychildmatters.gov.uk/aims/childrenstrusts/; accessed 2 December 2007.

Wanless, D. (2002) *Securing Our Future Health: Taking a Long-Term* View. HM Treasury, London.

Wanless, D. (2004) *Securing Good Health for the Whole Population*. HM Treasury, London.

Wanless, D. (2007) *Our Future Health Secured? A Review of NHS Funding and Performance*. King's Fund Publications, London.

Webster, C. and French, J. (2003) The cycle of conflict: the history of the public health and health promotion movements. In: *Debates and Dilemmas in Promoting Health* (eds. M. Sidell, L. Jones, J. Katz, A. Peberdy and J. Douglas). Palgrave Macmillan, London.

Whitehead, D. (2003) Evaluating health promotion: a model for nursing practice. *Journal of Advanced Nursing*, **41**(5), 490–8.

World Health Organization (1978) *Alma Ata Declaration*. http://www.righttohealthcare.org/Docs/DocumentsC.htm; accessed 12 December 2007.

World Health Organization (2000) *The Fifth Global Conference on Health Promotion: Bridging the Equity Gap*. http://www.who.int/healthpromotion/conferences/previous/mexico/en/hpr_mexico_report_en.pdf; accessed 12 December 2007.

World Health Organization (2005) *The Bangkok Charter: 6th Global Conference on Health Promotion*. http://www.who.int/healthpromotion/conferences/6gchp/bangkok_charter/en/index.html; accessed 12 December 2007.

Index